Daniel Lakell

Office of Okult

Probation.

112 W. Pennington St.

Tucson, Arizona

Pelican Book A695

New Horizons in Psychiatry

Peter Hays, who is Senior Lecturer in
Psychiatry at St George's Hospital,
London, was born in Wimbledon in 1927,
and educated at grammar schools. He
served with the Royal Engineers as a staff
sergeant from 1945 to 1948, and then went
to King's College, London, and St
George's Hospital where he qualified
in 1954. Besides St George's,
he has also worked at St Andrew's
Hospital, Northampton. He
does clinical, teaching, and research work
in about equal proportions, and has had
glimpses of psychiatry in both the U.S.A.
and the U.S.S.R.

Peter Hays, who lives with his family at
Wimbledon, also writes novels under a
pseudonym, to subsidize the pleasant
calling of academic medicine.

Peter Hays

New Horizons in Psychiatry

Penguin Books
Baltimore · Maryland

Penguin Books Ltd, Harmondsworth,
Middlesex, England
Penguin Books Inc., 3300 Clipper Mill Road,
Baltimore 11, Md, U.S.A.
Penguin Books Pty Ltd, Ringwood,
Victoria, Australia

First published 1964

Made and printed in Great Britain by
Cox and Wyman Ltd,
London, Reading, and Fakenham
Set in Monotype Imprint

Contents

Preface

In this book I have tried to outline the fast-expanding areas of psychiatric research, describing at the same time some of the recent work in this active branch of medicine. It has been my aim to avoid speculation, except when some hypothesis was needed to give order to a section. This bias in favour of factual accounts of work done, rather than notions about how things might be if one were only to look into them, has made me rely very much on articles and commentaries published in psychiatric journals and those of allied disciplines. Therefore, I am very content to say, this book is almost entirely a work of plagiarism and, since I have often been unable to better the phrases used by individual authors, is as much an anthology as a review of the field.

Apart from the general debt I owe to my colleagues, I wish to acknowledge the helpful comments of Professor D. Curran, and Sir Paul Mallinson, who read the whole of the original manuscript; psychiatrists who read over single chapters concerning subjects in which they had a special interest, included Professor E. Stengel (Sheffield), Dr A. Hoffer (Saskatchewan), Dr B. A. O'Connell (Broadmoor), and Dr H. Rollin (Horton Hospital). Mr T. E. Walsh (Neurosurgeon to St George's Hospital) kindly suggested modifications of the chapter on Neurosurgical Advances and Mr H. Gwynne Jones, the psychologist, read and made welcome suggestions about the chapters on Pavlov and Psychological Testing. Dr A. W. Nineham gave me invaluable assistance in compiling the chapter on new drugs. None of those named above necessarily endorses my views in this book and the responsibility for all errors is my own.

Introduction

It is customary to start any general account of psychiatry by enumerating the beds devoted to those with psychiatric illnesses, and though this is a rather unoriginal approach, the figures are so striking that mention of them must be made. About half of the hospital beds in use in a civilized country are usually occupied by psychiatric patients, most of them long-term and a high proportion of them schizophrenic. Psychiatric illnesses lead to mortality even in this country, and are the principal cause behind our 5,000 suicides per annum, to mention that mode of death alone. Psychological symptoms lie at the back of an uncertain but high proportion of the complaints of patients seen in general practice, particularly those patients who return again and again. But one of the main changes that has taken place in recent years is a new awareness of the extent of psychiatric disability and the need to reduce this by all possible means.

The scope of the illnesses regarded as psychiatric is as great as the volume of patients. Some illnesses have a definite and well-known organic basis, so that pathological changes can invariably be found at post-mortem examinations; some are the consequences of well-known biochemical aberrations; others are, or are thought probably to be, dependent on subtle alterations in complex biochemical equilibria; still others, the majority, are so poorly understood in the scientific sense of the word that the language of classical medicine has to be discarded and the processes described in mythological and metaphorical terms of mortifying ambiguity.

In this book much reference will be made to work that is recent or, though venerable, still incomplete: in writing of new directions it is necessary that some older orientations be established early on. So in the second half of this introduction I will give a brief history of early psychiatry and mental health in order to show how radical and striking the modern, altered approach is. In order to provide the reader with an idea of the span of psychiatry first, however, a short account of the diagnostic range of the subject and the commoner treatments of accepted usefulness will be given at this stage.

I shall first describe the troublesome but comparatively minor illnesses called psychoneuroses (including anxiety states, hysterical conversion syndromes, obsessive-compulsive neuroses, and phobic states) before turning to the psychoses, the most profound of the psychological disorders. Some psychoses, the functional psychoses, such as manic-depressive psychosis and schizophrenia, have no known pathological basis; while others, the organic psychoses, are associated with discernible changes in the patient's body, such as a brain tumour, senile ageing changes, and so on. I shall then touch upon a miscellany of conditions which sometimes come the psychiatrist's way, indicating how much or how little the psychiatrists are justifiably concerned in different instances.

Because these descriptions are simply introductory, and are expanded where necessary in later chapters, the psychiatrist who is reading the book out of idle curiosity may skip this section without loss, but the general reader with little specialist knowledge would be well advised to read it through because though many terms used in psychiatry have been borrowed from or assimilated into ordinary language, their technical meanings are not necessarily the same; and also because this book is concerned with a wider range of illness and treatment than is usually discussed when intelligent laymen light upon the topic of psychodynamics.

PSYCHONEUROSES (NEUROSES)

These illnesses are most easily understood by approaching them through a description of normal people. Everybody is subjected, from time to time, to stress, in the course of which he experiences anxiety. This normal phenomenon, anxiety, is central to the psychoneuroses, in which, however, its biological purpose of making us take avoiding action is no longer served. The universal emotion of anxiety is associated with restlessness and increase in muscular tone, and the heart and vascular system contribute to a generalized preparation for action; the pupils dilate, the hands tremble, and the palms and soles of the feet become damp. Victims of anxiety feel a need to move about, to act, to decide, and thus to end whatever dilemma they find themselves in; and the anxiety tends to increase until they are forced to a decision, whereupon, even if the decision is the wrong one, the anxiety falls away. Normally anxiety is dispelled by these mechanisms of making the mind up and dealing with the source of anxiety or moving rapidly away. The emotion of anxiety in its fully developed form is so unpleasant that we become skilled at taking preventive action at the first sign of a threat, thus avoiding, except in times of national upheaval or individual disaster, the extremes of anxiety known as panic. Anxiety may therefore be regarded as adaptive, in that it makes us individually and evolutionarily more suited to the world, encouraging us to avoid danger and trouble if we can, and deal with it if we cannot. (Under certain circumstances the normal human being comes up against difficulties that he obviously cannot avoid or deal with; then resignation supervenes and anxiety is prevented by auxiliary psychological mechanisms, such as dissociation. This is presumably how almost all murderers awaiting trial are able to eat well, sleep well, and gain weight, in spite of their un-enviable situation.)

The neurotic reacts badly or inappropriately to stress. Either he experiences more anxiety than most, or he experiences anxiety because of threats that he cannot identify. Having developed severe anxiety, he may fail entirely to deal with the problem, thus condemning himself to an increase of the emotion, or he may get rid of his anxiety by a means that leaves the source of it untouched and therefore builds up trouble for himself in the long run. Clinical examples will illustrate the effect of these misapplications of the anxiety mechanisms that are built into the central nervous system.

Some people are peculiarly anxiety-prone, experiencing

mild apprehension even in the face of minor troubles. They may be described as having an anxious personality. This, if extreme, may constitute one of the personality problems mentioned later, but does not necessarily lead to psychiatric modification; indeed, the anxious man may exploit his alertness and over-concern to improve his earning capacity: the tense and jumpy businessman is a familiar figure despite the value his profession places on appearing relaxed. Such a man may, under unusual strain, develop overt anxiety to a level that starts to reduce his efficiency. The tendency of anxiety to increase decisiveness has as a corollary certain disadvantages: for example, under the spur of anxiety decisions are taken only on the most obvious evidence, and unlikely or subtly reached decisions are automatically ruled out. This is biologically helpful in a physical emergency, but less appropriate to decisions that have to be taken about complicated policy or personnel matters. People of this kind are used to some anxiety and able to tolerate it well, but they may 'present' (a term which I shall use for coming to a doctor) with the psychoneurosis called an *anxiety state* if their tolerance is overcome by the severity of the symptoms or the length of time they have persisted.

Some patients develop severe anxiety not because they are specially prone to this reaction but because for some reason they are unable to recognize its source: it may be that a figure with whom a patient is forced into contact is someone whom he at once dislikes and is unable to admit he dislikes, like a new wife or a younger colleague and friend, who threatens to supplant him. Classically, the patient with an anxiety state is reckoned to have a complex, the consequence of repressed desires in early life, which causes symptoms in him years later; in practice, however, patients are usually found to have some rather mundane problem that is responsible for their symptoms, often obvious to all and of recent origin.

The patient with prolonged anxiety is uncomfortable, finds it difficult to get off to sleep, may be irritable and jumpy, and fatigues easily because of his muscular tension. If his stresses persist, or, proving permanent, cannot be accepted, his symptoms become clamorous.

It is at this stage that alternative, and neurotic, mechanisms may be called in to deal with the anxiety. One well-known method by which patients deal with the discomfort is to develop what are called *hysterical conversion symptoms*. Certain patients are able to fall ill in an apparently physical way when anxiety gets too much for them, and as a result their colleagues recognize that they are unable to deal with any problems that arise; such hysterical illnesses are commonly associated, at their onset, with a sharp reduction in the level of experienced anxiety, for the illness removes the need for any decision or action to be taken.

One well-known example of the hysterical group of illnesses is amnesia. The symptom of total loss of memory for name and address and much or all of the past is one which, if it were the consequence of damage to the brain, would necessarily include loss of the capacity to speak coherently and perform skilled movements; if a patient presents himself at a casualty department saying that he has lost his memory, then it may be confidently inferred that the illness is functional – is either hysteria or malingering. The distinction between hysteria and malingering cannot be confidently made – if the patient is lying about his memory he is malingering, but if he believes it, he is hysterical; only the patient can tell which is the case and sometimes even he is uncertain. Most hysterical amnesias clearly start off by being malingered: patients usually arrive without identifying documents in pocket or handbag, so it may be assumed that at the time they removed these their actions were purposive and consciously undertaken. Many such patients are escaping or trying to escape from the consequences of a crime or misdemeanour.

For a hysterical episode to take place, the patient must be somewhat primitive, and indeed there is a notable social and racial variation in the incidence of hysteria. If, as still occasionally happens, hysteria occurs in intelligent and psychologically sophisticated patients, it is often some other process, such as organic brain disease, that has reduced the patient's capacity for self-criticism. Subjectively comfortable though hysterical conversion syndromes are, they are inefficient methods of dealing with anxiety because they do nothing about the stress itself, and indeed, by introducing physical red herrings, distract both the patient's and the doctor's attention from the real threat. Therefore, unless the threat is removed by some chance, the conversion symptoms must be prolonged indefinitely, and even when the stress no longer operates it may be impossible for the patient, whether through pride or medical mismanagement, to relinquish the physical symptom.

Hysterical conversion symptoms tend to be produced by patients with what is called hysterical personality: a provocative and emotionally shallow personality, often with a theatrical and demonstrative façade. This relationship between personality and neurotic mechanism is not consistent, but occurs frequently enough to make it more than a chance finding.

Another type of personality, the obsessional personality, is prone, under certain types of stress, to develop an *obsessive-compulsive neurosis*. The obsessional person, or *anankast*, is inclined to be neat and orderly, parsimonious though capable of the hospitality required by local convention, conscientious to a greater extent than is necessary or comfortable, greatly taken with routine, uneasy about flouting traditional rules and superstitions, 'bowel-conscious', and given, particularly when tense, to the performance of harmless little rituals. He is a good person to have as a subordinate, an exacting colleague, and a critical superior, and he works best in a strictly hierarchical organization with precise job-delineation.

This kind of man is rendered uneasy both by disturbance of routine and by any impulses he may feel to depart from the dictates of his powerful conscience, while correspondingly the performance of a ritual cleansing or the conscientious discharge of a duty produce in him some diminution of his constant background anxiety and doubt. It is understandable, then, that any temptations he may feel to depart from his high principles will cause him great anxiety and that, since it is often impossible for him to consider or admit to himself the possession of wicked impulses, he may deal with this guilty anxiety in his usual way – by increasing the amount and frequency of his ritual behaviour. For example, if a man who always lathers and shaves himself twice and rinses his hands three times after going to the lavatory experiences a brief urge to commit adultery with his sister-in-law, this may be followed with an upsurge of minor ritualistic behaviour that persists until the memory of the taboo wish fades away. If he is unfortunate enough to experience the identical desire recurrently, or if it is persistent, the rituals become less efficacious in relieving his anxiety and may need to be repeated several times. When repetition of a tolerable kind becomes ineffective the resulting increases in frequency of the rituals and the time they consume make them become, in their turn, a source of unpunctuality and inefficiency, and therefore of fresh anxiety. Evidently, in this idealized case history, there is a point of no return, after which the anxiety secondary to the rituals causes more ritualistic activity to be indulged in, and even if the original source of anxiety is then dealt with in some way, the obsessive-compulsive state remains and continues to be self-propagating.

Phobic states seem to arise in a similar manner to obsessive-compulsive neuroses, when anxiety is focused on to an objectively neutral stimulus, commonly one with some special meaning for the patient or a general tendency to cause sub-threshold anxiety in most people, such as that associated with enclosed spaces. A patient, in this instance usually a woman, may become phobic about travel to an extent that causes her to be virtually confined to her home; other patients may be phobic about dogs, cats, bridges, heights, or other comparatively harmless (but often vaguely threatening) things. The patient's battle with the phobia diverts attention from the real source of the anxiety and the effects the phobia has on her life provide a separate and increasing complement of this basic emotion, with an inevitable tendency to progression.

It is a cardinal principle in psychiatry that causation is always multiple, including physical, psychological, and constitutional (meaning, approximately, inborn) part-causes, so that *treatment*, ideally aimed at eradicating the cause, is never unitary; but in the main psychoneuroses are satisfactorily managed by psychotherapy, a process of verbal interchange which aims at revising the patient's attitudes. Untreated, these illnesses show a natural tendency towards improvement, so that it is difficult to compare the effectiveness of the many different types of psychotherapy; if on the other hand, the type of treatment given is prolonged it is never certain whether psychotherapy or the passage of time led to the improvement that finally took place.

FUNCTIONAL PSYCHOSES

Psychosis is the term used to refer to a profound disease of the mind in which new symptoms, divorced in quality or degree from what is normally experienced, make an appearance or in which fundamental brain-functions, such as those concerned in the perception of the world, become disordered.

Some of the psychoses, to which reference will be made shortly, arise as the inevitable consequence of gross damage to the brain. In distinction from these *organic psychoses* there exist two important illnesses: schizophrenia and affective psychosis (including manic-depression), in which no organic changes are found, and which are subsumed under the general title of *functional psychoses*.

The word 'affect' is used in psychiatry, for reasons that have never been made clear to me, instead of the word 'mood'. *Affective psychoses* are those in which all alterations in mental function spring from a pathologically disordered mood. Thus the patient may be depressed or, much less commonly, elated, and all his symptoms are explicable on the basis of the mood change which itself, however, defies explanation. The elation (in *mania* and its lesser variant *hypomania*) and the depression arise from no apparent or adequate cause and persist in a way that normal emotions do not.

When depressed, the patient presents a picture of misery and helpless worry, and his mood has a genuine and affecting quality that moves the observer more even than evidence of severe physical pain (which those who have experienced both would prefer to suffer if given the choice). His conversation seems rational enough and rapport is excellent. The psychotic nature of the illness is evident in its arrival from nowhere or without adequate precipitation, its total unresponsiveness to all the measures that might be expected to cheer a person up, and the patient's partial or total loss of insight – he believes he is depressed because he is wicked, or because doom lies round the corner, or because he is bankrupt (if a businessman), due for court-martial (if in the services), or has lost his faith (if a priest). People who have experienced neither depression nor the privilege of treating depressed patients are inclined to believe that those who succumb to affective illness of this kind are inadequate individuals who cannot or, more likely, will not face up to things: the truth is rather the reverse. Most patients have received plenty of advice from relatives and friends to the effect that they should snap out of it, advice which is not only impossible to follow, this being the essence of the illness, but is peculiarly insulting in that it implies that the patient was too stupid to think up the plan himself. Depressed patients often express their surprise and gratitude that the psychiatrist does not in turn tell them to get a grip on themselves, but their main cause for contentment is the prompt effectiveness of the treatment available; relief of symptoms by psychiatric intervention does not alter the outcome, for this is one of recovery whether the patient is treated or not, but it speeds the recovery and may prevent weeks, months, or years of misery, despair, and unemployment.

The manic or the mildly manic patient, commonly called the hypomanic, is not so comfortable to treat as the patient in a depressed phase, because he is inclined to be argumentative, dictatorial, and haughty, in keeping with his elevated mood, and because he frequently feels far better than he ever has in his life before and cannot see why his relatives and doctors should be so deluded as to imagine that he needs treatment (his well-being is unfortunately often associated with gross prodigality and outspokenness, and the condition does in fact require correction despite its subjective advantages). In manic and hypomanic states treatment is also effective; usually the patient may be discharged within a very few weeks.

The importance of these illnesses lies in their high incidence, their tendency to relapse (i.e. to recur soon after treatment is finished), their tendency to later recurrence (fresh illnesses not uncommonly occurring from time to time throughout life), their complications, notably suicide, and the horrific nature of the experience of prolonged and hopeless depression. The good outlook and, lately, the effectiveness of therapy, have prevented as much time and effort being lavished on the causes of these illnesses as has been expended on schizophrenia, but the diseases are in many ways an easier research proposition than schizophrenia, because of the experimental advantages of the recurrent course of depressive states. In recurrent affective illness the patient's chemistry and abnormal psychology need not be compared with that of another, well, person, who may differ in all kinds of unpredictable ways; they may be compared with findings in the same patient when he is between illnesses.

In these classical depressions that occur without apparent cause, the depressions constitute episodes in the manic-depressive psychosis. Patients suffering from this condition have family histories of similar illnesses, and to a large extent the illness is genetically determined. Other types of severe depression may occur in patients without strong family histories of depressive illness (and, in particular, without evidence of episodes of elation) after such physical stresses as influenza-like illnesses, jaundice, head-injury, and the use of certain drugs. Psychological factors, apparently operating as non-specific influences rather than obviously comprehensible causes, and including bereavement (not necessarily of a well-loved relative) and long-standing anxiety, are often of importance in the causation of psychotic depressions and their analysis is of particular use in the prevention of relapse.

Treatment of the affective psychoses, whatever precipitates them, is primarily physical and pharmacological. Admission to hospital is often necessary to prevent the depressive from committing suicide or to obtain some control over the conduct of the hypomanic. Psychotherapy is an integral part of the management because it helps to stop the patient from relapsing, but the use of electricity or the new anti-depressive drugs is the principal treatment.

These illnesses leave no sequel of altered function.

The other great functional psychosis is called *schizophrenia*. This illness has a prevalence somewhat higher than that of

Schizophren

classical affective psychoses; though only about 8 per 1,000 of the population develop schizophrenia, and less new cases of schizophrenia are seen at consulting sessions than new cases of depression the illness transcends the affective psychoses in importance because it has a natural tendency to progress insidiously and inexorably. The symptoms of this illness are very varied, but all the clinical sub-types of schizophrenia have general features in common: usually young people are affected, once ill they show an inclination to withdraw, and as the illness progresses the personality, though not the intellect, shows signs of dilapidation. The schizophrenic's inner life becomes of more concern to him than objective reality, against which he does not check his ideas, so that he shows what has been described as 'a characteristic diminution of the quality of critical appraisal'.

These general statements apart, individual schizophrenics also have a selection of more dramatic symptoms: some, the *paranoid schizophrenics*, are notably hallucinated (perceiving – usually hearing – things when there is nothing there) and deluded (possessed of false beliefs of a fixed and pathological type); the *catatonic schizophrenics* may also be hallucinated and deluded but principally display symptoms of disordered muscular activity – moving stiltedly, too slow, or too fast; the *hebephrenic schizophrenics* mostly show a failure of logical thoughts, and the *simple schizophrenics* mainly a negative picture of withdrawal and inertia. These sub-groupings, though not essential to a grasp of the nature of the illness, highlight the variety of symptoms of schizophrenia. They are best seen in early (acute) schizophrenics, for as time goes by the rather uniform condition of *chronic* schizophrenia supervenes and the distinction between the sub-groups becomes blurred and doubtful.

Treatment of acute illnesses depends mainly on drugs, particularly the phenothiazine type of tranquillizer. Other measures are used for convenience and the benefit of particular symptoms, and the patient's needs for explanation and support are filled by psychotherapy, usually of a non-exploratory kind. Insulin coma therapy is now seldom used, though available in a few hospitals for the convenience of doctors who cling to it still (and who may be right to do so). Once a patient's illness, having failed to respond more than temporarily to treatment, becomes chronic, the management alters. Though drugs and other characteristically medical measures may still be used, the therapeutic endeavours are mainly concerned with training and socialization. Vigorous régimes of cooperative occupation seek to turn the patient from his inner life to reality. This treatment is not curative and, despite high discharge figures at the present time, does not necessarily fit the patient for the outside world; but it saves the chronic schizophrenic from the oddities, mannerisms, and personal degradation that were the rule before the war. The prognosis for untreated schizophrenia is poor, with a recovery rate, probably, of less than one quarter. The outlook with present-day treatment is moderately good for a first acute attack if the patient's original (*premorbid*) personality was a normal one, but there is much variability in the results reported today, so that no hard-and-fast odds can be given, while as yet we do not know what the long-term results of drug therapy will be.

THE ORGANIC PSYCHOSES

The *organic psychoses* are found in the presence of known or confidently inferred chemical or physical abnormality. The epileptic twilight states, fugues, and psychoses are associated with electro-encephalographic findings of a specific kind. Some, the common deliria, occur in the course of serious physical illness or after head injury or other brain damage. Others may be the consequence of infections of the brain or its coverings, or intoxication with drugs or industrial poisons. The foregoing are the more acute and temporary of the organic psychoses, and produce, in general, a reduction in the level of consciousness (varying from mild difficulty in grasp to deep coma) and failures of memory. Epileptic psychoses may cause vivid hallucinations with delusional ideas that are reminiscent of those seen in schizophrenia (which may be distinguished only with some difficulty). Delirious patients become uncertain of what is going on round them, misinterpret what they see and hear, and see and hear things that are not there, therefore becoming deluded about what is happening to them; they become over-active and restless, whether through fear of the abnormal phenomena they perceive or for other less comprehensible reasons, and are disorientated (do not know where they are or what time it is). Treatment is that of the causal condition, where this can be dealt with, and is otherwise aimed at relieving the symptoms and reducing the exhaustion produced by over-activity.

The more chronic of the organic psychoses include the late consequences of syphilis and the damage caused by brain tumours or other space-occupying lesions within the skull, but for the most part they are the outward signs of degenerative processes, particularly those of senility. Though treatment of these chronic illnesses is aimed at the cause if this can be found, investigations seldom disclose treatable abnormalities, and the patients show a gradually increasing loss of intellectual ability (called *dementia*) accompanied by a disintegration of personality, with death usually supervening after a year or two.

Apart from these more or less specific illnesses, psychiatrists also deal with a variety of miscellaneous conditions. Some of these are of note because they may be evidence of serious underlying psychotic or psychoneurotic illness rather than because they are principally caused by psychological factors or are mainly treatable by psychological means. Examples of these states include the *addictions*, whether to drugs or alcohol, in which certain biochemical and metabolic changes of an ill-defined kind attend the development of addiction and which, though there may be no causal psychological anomalies concerned, have the characteristics of a true illness once they are established. Thus when he treats an alcohol addict, a psychiatrist looks first for underlying psychiatric illness and if, as is usually the case, he fails to find it, he then treats his patient as any doctor would, applying no psychological techniques unknown to a good general physician. In this situation his initial function is one of ruling out true psychiatric illness, and his later work, though equally skilled, is not strictly an integral part of his speciality.

Similarly the psychiatrist is often involved in criminological work. His function here, as in addiction, was at one time confined to ruling out overt and definite psychiatric illness; but unlike the addict, the criminal who is free from psychiatric disorder does not show another, non-psychiatric illness, only a disorder of conduct.

During work with criminals and delinquents and, to a lesser extent, with alcohol addicts, psychiatrists came to see and recognize certain types of personality that, being possessed by those who sought oblivion or caused trouble, were considered unenviable or undesirable. These individuals – not qualitatively different from the rest of the public but endowed with attributes that made for trouble for themselves or others – were recognized as having what are called *personality deviations* and some of them, notably those whose deviations led to anti-social activity of a persistent kind, were called psychopaths. They are distinct from the psychotic and most of the psychoneurotic patients seen, but no clear-cut distinction exists between them and the rest of the public.

Thus, by way of summary revision, since these distinctions are not easy to grasp when described at the present pace, the patient who comes to the doctor because he is as he is and has always been, has a *personality disorder*; the patient who comes because under certain stresses he has, in view of his particular personality, reacted with comprehensible but inefficient anxiety symptoms (or some substitute for these), has a *psychoneurosis*; while the patient who comes because his mind has started to show severe disorders of function such as memory-failure or some loss of contact with what is real, has a *psychosis*.

Psychiatry is commonly said to be concerned with the study, diagnosis, and treatment of illnesses in which psychological factors are pre-eminent in the symptoms displayed or the causation of those symptoms. At one time this would have been a complete definition; psychiatry is what psychiatrists do, and that is what they did. Today, however, whether they wish it or not, psychiatrists do more. Having excluded illness proper from individuals at the fringe of psychiatry they may still be requested or expected to provide assistance, and often do so.

For the addict much of this help still falls within the clinical frame of reference – an illness exists and is treated; poorly treated, it is true, but along orthodox medical lines. When it comes to the management of personality disorders and, still more markedly, that of persons whose conduct has outraged the public (such as normal criminals) the psychiatrist is no longer treating ill people but assisting the poorly adjusted to fit in or to be less unhappy. This is a far cry from the usual medical process of determining the nature of an illness and dealing with it in such a way as to return the organism to its premorbid state, and resembles education more than traditional treatment.

Some psychiatrists have welcomed this extension of their speciality. They may feel that not only is the study of the normal valuable as a guide to abnormality but, in agreement with Freud, that from normal psychology spring all the functional psychiatric illnesses that are seen in clinical practice, so that no illness differs except in degree from what is normally found, and all conditions seen, no matter how nearly they correspond to normality, are grist to the psychiatric mill. Others seek to re-establish limits corresponding to those found in other branches of medicine, where a patient wasted by disease is treated, but a puny man of the same weight and strength is not; attempts to set formal boundaries to the speciality in this way, though a healthy reaction to exaggerated claims that have been made by psychiatrists of a generation or two ago, founder on the psychoneuroses, the most severe of which constitute undoubted illnesses, while the most mild blend with the normal worries and defences of everyday life. The extent to which psychiatrists let their work and interest expand is of no great importance provided it is realized that the exclusively medical nature of their work ends as they turn to personality deviations and the study of such normal variations as the commoner perversions. Only if they are expected to deal with these conditions in the usual medical way, by drugs or some other putative cure, or if they mistake their interest for outright ownership and expect other workers to take second place in their management, need the divisions cause confusion.

(II) THE ALTERING APPROACH

In the first, exploratory stages of a scientific study the greater part of the work done is descriptive. The early psychiatrists made accounts of their patients' symptoms with both scientific and practical motives. The logical extension of description is classification, and they hoped to bring some order to the chaotic ranks of the insane by consideration of the symptoms with which a series of patients had presented, expecting that an examination of their case histories would enable certain categories of symptom-complex to be extracted and labelled diseases. Psychiatric patients, unfortunately for this exercise, have only a very few symptoms between them, and the most dramatic and obvious of these, such as delusions and hallucinations, are not characteristic of any specific disease; so that none of the old-fashioned classifications is now of interest except to the medical historian.

As before and since, ignorance did not prevent psychiatrists of that time, together with any others who felt the need or the capacity, from postulating theories about mental malfunction. The ideas put forward reflected the morality of the day more than the clinical observation that had been made, and none of the fanciful schemata could hope to point the way to beneficial treatment. (There was one chance exception: certain failures of nervous function, such as epilepsy and what is now called schizophrenia, were thought to be due to masturbation – noted as taking place in patients under observation but thought to be rare in the unafflicted – and bromides were given in an attempt to reduce sexual drive; these salts are both sedative and anti-epileptic and therefore brought about some benefit. The partial effectiveness of bromides was taken, in a manner that still offers a warning to experimental physicians, to demonstrate the correctness of the theory that suggested them.)

The practical purpose behind the elucidation of symptoms was the pointers these provided to treatment. Nowadays the eradication of pain or of the patient's awareness that some pathological process is under way by the use of symptomatic treatment is regarded almost invariably as a sign of failure unless it is instituted merely for stop-gap purposes. Thus the patient with a painful abdomen is rarely given morphine or a similar drug until the cause of the pain has been determined and treatment of a radical kind either put under way or recognized as impossible. An example from general medicine is given because psychiatry is still at a comparatively rude level, and much of the sedative and other treatment offered to psychiatric patients is aimed solely at reducing current discomfort, without the expectation of permanent benefit. In the eighteenth and nineteenth centuries medical and psychiatric treatment was virtually restricted to piecemeal reduction of the patient's complaints and much regard was therefore paid to individual symptoms, though the remedies available for their amelioration were seldom of any intrinsic value.

Because most of the theories were obviously unlikely (to all but their perpetrators) and since the treatment was mostly ineffective, the leaders of the speciality cast about for alternative methods of investigation.

In the middle of the nineteenth century one type of study was proving its general worth. Cholera was common in London at that time, and a survey of its incidence showed that some areas had many cases and others few; when the different factors operating upon the two populations – heavily affected and lightly affected – were examined it was found that they derived their water from separate sources. Substitution of another water supply for that associated with the cholera epidemic ended the outbreak concerned. This is a well-known and classical example of the *epidemiological method* and its practical application: the incidence of a disease is determined and where different incidences are found, an explanation of the variation is sought in the differing circumstances of the people concerned. Since it is not always necessary for the precise cause of the disease to be known (indeed, in the example given, it was thirty years before the cholera vibrio was identified) for preventive action to be taken, the epidemiological method had obvious application in psychiatry, where causes were obscure, treatment ineffectual, and prevention seemed the only hope.

Victorian psychiatrists undertook some comparative epidemiological studies which, though primitive, were sensible
in their design. Daniel Hack Tuke in 1878 wrote a book called
*Insanity in Ancient and Modern Life, with chapters on
Prevention*, commending it especially to 'those who may
reasonably suspect that they have the seeds of madness sown in
their own constitution, or are conscious of a tendency to irregu-
lar mental action' and thereby, one surmises, riveting the attention of a substantial section of the public. He tried to correlate
the types of insanity described in Israel, Ancient Greece, and
Imperial Rome with the lives of the Jews, the Greeks, and the
Romans as far as he could judge them, comparing all these findings with his knowledge of contemporary England. After prolonged analysis he was led to advise self-control, moderation,
and continence as the best hope of preservation of the shaky
mind, the qualities named being those most obviously lacking
in the epochs under review. The quality of the data available to
him meant that, apart from frightening his more rational
readers, he could accomplish nothing, but the method was
sound and might have been further pursued had it not been for
independent developments in medical science.

Soon after this book was published the grand era of the
bacteriologists and pathologists opened. Broad studies of illness
were put on one side as organism after organism was found.
Koch discovered, described, and named the causative micro-
organism of cholera all within two weeks in 1883, and he and his
colleagues conducted a kind of triumphal march, not without
battle casualties for the bacteriologists, through the infectious
diseases. The science of pathology even breached the walls of
the mental hospitals, elucidating the illness called General
Paralysis of the Insane, so that not only the general hospitals
but the asylums seemed about to benefit and a wave of optimism,
not the first or the last, swept over psychological medicine. The
bathos of the sequel in psychiatry provides a corrective to an
overdramatic summary of this epoch, for no further application
of the new knowledge was found.

Nevertheless, the new dimensions provided by pathology –
the study of disease and its processes instead of simply the

sick person of here and now – enlarged the view of the psychiatrist, making him look at the way in which symptoms arose: this development owes most of its success to the genius of Sigmund Freud, whose work so overshadows that of others that when the word psychopathology is used it is of his constructs that the student most commonly thinks.

Freud, over a number of years, produced a system of psychology and psychopathology that was all-embracing and internally consistent. Unlike the psychologies of the philosophers and early experimenters, it was derived from information given by patients and it promised wide therapeutic applications. The psychopathology was complicated but comprehensible, and some of the propositions, for example, that the unconscious obeyed different laws from the logical and reality-based conscious, and that emotional complexes associated with buried memories could modify responses to current events, had a great and lasting effect on practical psychiatry. Freud, in his writings and reasonings, initially gave due regard to inherited predispositions, but his main concern was with the influences of early life, in which he ultimately came to see the principal – almost the only – arbiters of the fate of the personality.

Apart from the new insights he gave his fellow-psychiatrists, Freud brought about many other changes: his work was accepted by the intelligentsia and became part of the fashionable conversational repertoire. Patients came to regard him as their prototypical psychiatrist and his methods as ideal, with all other approaches judged by the nearness with which they approximated to psychoanalysis; indeed, they still often use the word 'psychoanalysis', which strictly refers only to the Freudian method of treatment, interchangeably with 'psychiatry' or 'psychotherapy'. His work, by promising hope of cure in a field where no successful treatment was possible or in sight, produced some much-needed optimism. His frank discussion of sexual matters and childish passions did much to sweep away the hypocrisy of his cultural milieu. By stating a comprehensive philosophy, he brought hope of certainty to a world becoming sceptical of old dogma, and by translating the disturbing notion of insanity into commonplace terms and indicating the connexion between everyday and psychotic thinking seemed to reduce a mystery to the status of yet another scientific problem solved.

His popular influence persists; even today educated patients may expect to be asked about their dreams, or stretched out on a couch, or questioned closely about their earliest memories of incestuous passions, or requested to free-associate, none of which is commonly done. In the arts, particularly literature, psychoanalytical formulations and symbols are frequently utilized for their supposedly universal truth and recognizability.

In European psychiatric practice the best of Freud's work – that which has stood the test of experience and usefulness – is incorporated into the general body of knowledge. Some, understandably now that so much more work has been done on the same topics, has not stood up to the tests of time. A proportion, the most speculative and fanciful, is forgotten except when a stick is needed with which to beat the psychoanalysts when, as still regrettably happens, arguments unnecessarily arise. The weightiest theoretical objections to psychoanalytical doctrine lie in its non-scientific nature; every scientific statement should be and indeed, by definition, *is* concerned with possible experiment or observable processes, and some of Freud's dicta do not conform to this requirement, so that their complete acceptance has been described by some critics as smacking of religious rather than scientific conviction.

In the United States the body of doctrine, as a totality, was better received (there are more psychoanalysts practising in Philadelphia alone than in the whole of the United Kingdom) and it is still the mainspring of much of the clinical work and research in that country, though there are signs that its attraction for postgraduate psychiatric residents is waning. The reasons for the warmer welcome given to psychoanalysis in America are not altogether clear, but psychoanalysis requires a supply of well-to-do clients, to whom it can offer a patient educational and learning experience, and it gives some intellectual and emotional guidance and support of an authoritarian kind, similar to that rendered to the potential convert by Roman Catholicism, to patients whose previous values may have been discarded, along with other heavy baggage, during an arduous social climb. The success of orthodox Freudian psychoanalysis in the United States means that its practice must fill a real need, and there is no doubt that the quality of the psychotherapy is commonly very high, for the calibre of their psychoanalysts is formidable: but its quasi-theological nature means that such pockets as survive the rigorous assessments of efficacy that are now in vogue may well do so as offshoots of the main psychiatric growth.

Great men, particularly fluent ones working in a sphere where not much is known and everyone is looking for a lead, frequently suffer from their disciples. Freud, by concentrating on active, dynamic mental processes rather than the description and codification of sets of symptoms, substituted verbs for adjectives in psychiatry and took us from one era to another, but the over-valuing of his intuitions and surmises has had a stultifying effect in recent years. As will be seen, this effect was in part the consequence, not of his more doubtful doctrine or exotic explanations, but of the general acceptance of his insistence on the overriding importance in psychiatric illness of sexual and parental traumata inflicted before the age of five.

Some of the psychiatrists who followed Freud simply expanded his work, or stressed certain aspects of early experience, occasionally setting up minor schools of their own. Melanie Klein concentrated her attention on the very early period of late infancy and pre-oedipal childhood, while Anna Freud undertook the examination of defence mechanisms.

One psychiatrist, Carl Jung, departed from Freud's ideas in a rather grand way, but his work soon became more redolent of philosophical discourse than of scientific writing, and today a psychiatrist reads his books more for background education than technical assistance.

The last of the central triumvirate, Adler, viewed the personality and the personality-reactions called neuroses as the outcome of a struggle for power and domination and believed that men strove constantly to deny or to compensate for deep feelings of inferiority. His ideas, like those of all the great psychological theorists of this era, provided his readers with some illuminating insights, but they received less lasting attention than those of Freud and Jung because they could only explain a fraction of the behaviour patterns found in man. Nevertheless, they included a radical change of orientation. Adler recognized that the current events and interreactions of a person's life were of the greatest importance in determining how he acted, and rejected the views of those, of whom Freud was the exemplar, who believed that all was decided at the mother's breast or knee. His work thus represented a reversal of the trend towards regarding the psychology of the patient independently of his life-situation or day-to-day emotional involvements, and was at once a reversion to older views about the effects of society on man and a forerunner of a revival of interest in what has come to be called social psychiatry.

While Freud's work had been dominating the scene, setting off its intellectual and moral fireworks, psychiatrists in the mental hospitals had been steadily working away, trying to diagnose their patients. A general scheme of classification had been introduced by Kraepelin at the turn of the century, based not only on the patient's symptoms but on the outcome of his untreated disease, and this was steadily refined and modified. As a consequence, patients could usually be declared either organic, schizophrenic, manic-depressive or suffering from a minor mental illness such as a neurosis, and a prognosis of sorts could be offered. The reader will recall that Hack Tuke's epidemiological work foundered on lack of data, and this was not entirely because he could not know the prevailing social conditions in historical times with any accuracy; the first requirement of any epidemiological study is that the prevalence of the illness under review should be determined, and Tuke's ignorance of diagnosis would have made any attempt at an epidemiological survey even of his own time abortive because he had no means of separating the several psychiatric illnesses one from the other.

One condition, the mental state assumed to be associated with successful suicide, could be studied with fair accuracy because of its public and reportable nature, except where religious considerations and sympathy for the relatives led doctors to certify the cause of death falsely. Suicide has always been regarded with fascination and horror, and when its study was first undertaken on a large scale it was the social aspect of the abdication that was most closely examined, since suicide, with its rejection of the group's rules and demonstration of inadmissible despair, constitutes the greatest of the social affronts that an individual can provide. Working in the nineteenth century, Durkheim made a revealing study of this catastrophe: he found, *inter alia*, that suicide was commoner among Protestants than Catholics, regardless of their environment, and he connected a greater incidence of suicide with failure of group-identification. Though this work remained isolated for some time because other conditions were not, for the moment, accurately ascertainable, it set the style for future surveys, most of which have inquired into the social circumstances of the individuals affected rather than their innate psychological patterns.

This large-scale type of survey is a far cry from the prolonged examination of a few lucid and cooperative patients with subtle psychological imbalance, but a short account will be given of the present state of knowledge about suicide although no more than the most sketchy of pictures can be obtained of the suicides' mental state since the great majority are not psychiatric patients.

In many parts of the world suicide is on the increase. It is one of the major causes of death, killing annually almost as many as the motor-vehicle. A peak is found in the spring and early summer, at which time severe psychiatric illnesses are also more common, but mental illness in suicides is only found as a major cause in about one third, while many are found at autopsy to have severe physical illness. Suicide is less common in some of the primitive communities that have fragmentarily been reported on than it is in more civilized states, and commoner in towns than the country; the bigger the town, the higher the rate. It has no association with unemployment and it is negatively correlated with poverty, being rather more likely to occur in the upper social classes; it does have some correlation with new poverty, that is to say, with economic failure, and with social unrest. When social solidarity is high, as in wartime, suicides are less frequent, and, conversely, social disorganization is commonly reported in the milieu of the successful suicide. More than two thirds of these un-fortunates give some kind of warning of their intention (the unsubstantial notion that those who say they are going to, won't, is one of the costlier pieces of folk-lore) and many of the suicide notes indicate a real wish not to die.

The author himself treats individual patients and has no great wish to undertake long-range work of this kind, but readily admits that the result of the surveys is that there is more solid knowledge about suicide than about all the psychoneuroses put together. Furthermore – and this is a universal characteristic of present-day social studies – the data suggests many more urgent questions than its answers. Research into successful suicide is limited by the death of the principal, but obviously many of those who killed themselves were not so much success-ful suicides as attempts that in some way went wrong. E. Stengel followed up a series of patients who attempted suicide and survived, and his findings rounded out those of previous workers and gave impetus to a flurry of research on this aspect of the problem.

Those who attempt to kill themselves but survive constitute a different, though overlapping, population from those who die. Suicides are mainly older men, while those who attempt it are a younger group of whom the majority are female. The lower social classes are over-represented in those who attempt suicide, in contrast to the findings among suicides. Though attempts are very frequent, at least eight times as common as suicide itself, most deaths occur at the first try, and in spite of the fact that fresh attempts are not uncommon only a small proportion, probably less than ten per cent, of those who try and fail, ultimately kill themselves.

The suicide attempt, then, is not just a failed suicide: it is an attempt to communicate distress, as a last warning to society that help is needed. Once the attempt has been made the impor-tant figures in the patient's circle usually take some notice, and even those patients who make further serious attempts seldom do so until they have had time to note the effects of the first.

This is not to say that most of the attempts are not 'genuine' or are simply attention-seeking: the patient often courts death, giving to the episode the character of a trial by ordeal, and those fatalities whose warnings were emphatic and whose last notes yearned for life are the unlucky ones. Since the survivors are both treatable and available for interview, this kind of study is not confined to gross surveys of large numbers, but can ultimately focus on particular aspects of the mental state shown by the earlier work as liable to be of crucial interest. It is therefore capable of almost indefinite expansion.

Similar surveys have been undertaken of other illnesses, particularly schizophrenia, and the social circumstances of the patients noted. Schizophrenia, too, is more common in town than country, occurs more frequently in the unmarried than the 'ever-married' (those who, whatever their present civil status, have been married at one time) and seems to be associated with social isolation of some kind. Since 1964 all 'first admissions' (with basic data of a biological and diagnostic kind) have been collected statistically in this country, and it is to be hoped that manipulation of the data will produce helpful material. To some extent the usefulness of the method is still limited by the absence of great diagnostic uniformity; and standardization of criteria, a process that is under urgent review today, will be of great benefit.

The reader will discern that there are more profound distinctions to be drawn between the epidemiological research method and the individual-centred method than simply the inclusion in the former of the social characteristics of the patient's environment which, indeed, are incidental to the whole. The research done on individual patients is time-consuming and the data are subjectively obtained; such generalizations as can be made are therefore built on a small number of patients, not necessarily a homogeneous group and bearing no known relationship to the population to which generalization must refer. The generalizations are also heavily coloured by the researcher's presuppositions, of which he himself is not necessarily aware. Research on large groups, on the other hand, starts with the collection of objective and emotionally neutral material and only goes on to more detailed work when repeated correlations make generalizations impossible to avoid; it proceeds from the general to the particular. Evidently, as a scientific method, it has more chance of success, provided that it is not limited artificially to surveys of populations without following through on small groups of individuals.

This is not to say that the workers in the field of social studies have not their own preconceptions. The aim of research into medical subjects is almost always directly or indirectly to improve treatment and it is implicit in the work and the explanations that are put forward that some pathological social conditions, by favouring the emergence of individual pathology in the form of, say, suicide, provide a means of manipulating the environment beneficially if their exact nature can be ascertained. The flavour of this work and the rationalization of its results today is almost purely sociological: to take one example, the decrease in suicides and suicide attempts in wartime is invariably ascribed to increased social cohesion in time of national stress. This is in accordance with axioms of descriptive group psychology but alternative explanations abound; wars give the opportunity for much uninvestigated carelessness and high accident rates, and there is evidence that those who are suicidally inclined are notably more accident-prone; the suicide rate in Japan rose sharply after the war, but only if the forty *kamikaze* pilots who blew up each week are left out of the calculations and the selfless defenders of the Pacific islands ignored altogether.

The preoccupation of workers in this field with social factors has led them to take a look at the problem from a new angle. If illness depends for much of its incidence as well as its form on the social surroundings, then illness should vary with social class. Some research teams, therefore, instead of looking at the social circumstances surrounding various illnesses have stepped through the looking-glass and inquired into the variation in illnesses seen in the different social classes. The results, though unexplained, are astonishing. Classes are usually enumerated so as to avoid the emotional overtones of the everyday adjectives (lower, upper, etc), I being the professional class, III the skilled workers, and V the unskilled workers, with Classes II and IV intermediate; and it is found that the incidence of practically all the major mental illnesses is strikingly higher in the lowest class (V) than any other. The incidence (the rate at which new cases occur) of schizophrenia is five times as high in Class V as it is in Class I in some areas, while because of the poor outlook of Class V schizophrenics the prevalence (the actual number of people suffering from an illness at one time) may be nine times as great. Upper class psychotics frequently suffer from depressive illnesses but even this disease, once regarded as the perquisite of the able and effective, may be more frequent in its absolute incidence in Class V. Organic psychoses, including the senile psychoses, are also much more common in Class V subjects. Hollingshead and Redlich, whose work on this topic has been freely paraphrased here, write: 'Lower-class living appears to stimulate the development of psychotic disorders. We infer that the excess of psychoses from the poorer area is a product of the life conditions entailed in the lower socio-economic strata of the society.' This statement, though plausible and reflecting their motivation for doing the work, leaves the question of the subject's original endowments out of the picture; though it is not unlikely that the position a person holds in the class structure is dependent more on his potential than his origins as such, and that his diseases may arise because of innate weakness rather than the rigours of tenement life.

The medical concern with current and ameliorable traumata rather than endowment is partly due to a feeling that the endowment is fixed and any study of it, no matter how successful, must be therapeutically sterile. This is, of course, not the case. The genetic complement cannot be altered but the effects of faulty genes can be cancelled out in some illnesses – in diabetes, depression, phenylpyruvic oligophrenia (described in Chapter 12), and so on – and will become modifiable in others in time. Genetic studies arouse some antagonism also because of the manner in which the results seem to deny the importance of environmental influences, in which psychiatrists have a vested interest, but in fact, if correctly interpreted, most of the researches into psychiatric genetics have highlighted the over-whelming relevance of psychological and other stimuli.

Medical geneticists are well served by twins for reliable data and (if they can find enough pairs with illnesses) rapid answers: twins are either identical, with exactly the same genes, or frater-nal, with no more genetic or physical resemblance than brothers. In the research done on twins, the incidence of non-infective illnesses occurring in one of the members of each pair of twins is determined in the others. If an illness occurs with equal fre-quency in twins whether they are identical or fraternal, then environmental factors, being approximately the same for both, are likely to be mainly responsible. If on the other hand, the identical twins show a much higher concordance for the illness under review, then genetic factors are likely to be primarily concerned in its causation. By way of illustration of the results obtained, if schizophrenia occurs in one twin then his twin, if identical, has more than eight chances out of ten of developing the illness. On the other hand, if his twin is fraternal, or non-identical, his chances of succumbing to the process are small and no more than those of any other brother. Genetic data, particu-larly the finding just quoted, are often used when the efforts of psychiatrists to modify the schizophrenic's illness by psycho-logical means are being decried, while some clinicians, seeing in the 80:20 proportion provided by the geneticists a declaration that genes are four times as important as environmental factors in deciding whether the illness arises, have hotly attacked the methods and even the honesty of those concerned in psycho-genetics. In fact, of course, the interesting finding is that nearly 20 per cent of the identical twins of schizophrenics do not develop the illness; since their environments are virtually iden-tical and their genetic endowments are completely identical, this can only mean that whether or not a definite biologically founded predisposition to schizophrenia becomes the overt illness depends on the most subtle psychological or physical differ-ences in nurture.

Genetic work, like epidemiological applications in psychiatry, awaited some diagnostic consistency before it could be usefully undertaken. Once under way, however, it fed back information to the diagnosticians. Assistance is given in the classification of the psychoneuroses, of which some, such as obsessional neurosis, have a large hereditary component, while others, such as hysterical conversion states, have not and are therefore environmentally determined and, as such, likely to respond more easily to psychotherapeutic and other similar measures.

The reader will recall that the work of the pathologists and the academic psychologists had little to offer the clinical psychiatrists in the early years. While the psychiatric studies described so far were going on, both these branches of biological science were developing independently, and from time to time new methods produced by pathologists (and later, the biochemists) and psychologists were given a trial in psychiatric work. The increasing subtlety and precision of the techniques used led eventually to some practical and theoretical advances, while at the same time the advent of specific treatments in psychiatry, almost entirely as a consequence of a combination of chance and inspiration, led to an increase in the orderliness of the subject and its respectability as a branch of therapeutic science. These topics are discussed fully later in the book, but are mentioned here for the sake of continuity.

The new knowledge about the subject gave a death-blow to any hopes of a single, comparatively simple system of psychopathology: there is no panacea in psychiatry. The recognition that no logical explanation of the most severe psychological illnesses in terms of normal psychology or brain function could be offered led to acceptance of the necessity for a cooperative assault – in which practitioners in several disciplines would take part – on the problems disclosed by work already done. Because of the stress laid on personal psychodynamics by the Freudian school and those most influenced by the general theories of psychoanalysis, those who looked at the social rather than the individual characteristics of illness came to form a sub-speciality, calling themselves social psychiatrists. This artificial polarity, precipitated by Freud's work and the reaction against it, is bridged by general clinical psychiatrists, the majority in this country, who utilize what knowledge they can derive from not only the analytical and social psychiatrists but all the other disciplines whose work in any way impinges on theirs. Social psychiatry annexes to itself many different kinds of study, and thanks to its appeal and energetic pursuit many areas of human conduct are being explored as never before. Apart from the population surveys by nationally organized medical statisticians and the environmental correlations with diagnosis already mentioned, the sub-speciality is closely investigating the interaction of community and personality and the social aspects of treatment, particularly in order to find which social environments are associated, whether causally or not, with high recovery or relapse rates.

Attempts to do cross-cultural surveys to determine how illness varies with cultural background are usually baulked by the difficulty of ascertaining the illness rates in backward and underdoctored countries, and, complementarily, by the failure of present-day descriptive techniques to distinguish certainly between the sociology of civilized societies with differing incidences of psychiatric illness but broadly similar social organizations; such preliminary findings as there are, it is interesting to note, do not seem to support the feeling, to which many psychiatrists constantly hark back, that the savage is not only nobler but saner and in many ways healthier: psychosis-rates fall as societies move forward, and even duodenal ulcers, so long ascribed to the stress of modern civilization (strangely regarded as greater than it used to be when death, exploitation, disease, and poverty lurked round every corner) now seem to be lessening of their own accord. No experience in life is now immune from the social psychiatrists' interested examination: refugees, the bereaved, those awaiting operation, those settling into a New Town, and even those awaiting the end in a concentration camp are liable to find a psychiatrist (in the last instance, a fellow-prisoner) noting down their reactions for later publication in a learned journal. Social psychiatry is at present the most expansive and financially well-endowed of the psychiatric fields of action.

During the writing of this chapter the imposition of some kind of order on the sequence of researches and insights that led to the state of psychiatry as it existed during the post-war years has been possible with no more than a modicum of distortion and suppression. But the last ten years have seen such an explosion in scientific work of all kinds and such an immense increase in psychiatric research that the precarious coherence of this chapter would be threatened by any attempt to continue it as a sequential narrative, and the substance of the rest of the book deals with the various ways in which the new work has built on or demolished the old. This introductory section would not be complete, however, without a short discourse on what may ultimately be, for psychiatry, the most significant development in science, the application of which to psychiatric thought will one day provide us with new vocabularies and techniques.

Before the war the different branches of science were, to a great extent, separate. Communication between one scientist and another, even one working in a related field, was uncertain, and there was some concern about over-specialization and intellectual solitude. Nevertheless, there were aspects of all studies that were held in common: these related to the inter-actions of parts, the maintenance of equilibria and methods of control. For example, a thermostat had something in common with appetite, both switching on and off in accordance with information received from that which they were intended to affect; both had the same thing in common with a governor on an engine, and with an automatic pilot. The thermostat and the governor are comparatively simple devices, but in order to make an automatic pilot, or any other complex control device, the mathematics of control mechanisms had to be worked out.

The practical purposes for using these control devices were provided by war, but the conditions for their introduction on a large scale had existed for some years. The main aim of early engineers had been the provision of ample power, its control being left to men. Though mechanical power did not exist in abundance everywhere at the start of the Second World War, when most armies still relied largely on horse-drawn transport, its use in certain arms had increased to the point where the inefficiency of man (bred for other tasks in his long evolution) as a controller had started to show up. It was difficult for him to hold a fast-moving plane on target and, if he was on the ground, difficult for him to follow the plane with his gun.

The early work was assisted by half-forgotten calculations of mathematicians of previous generations, but was for the most part impressively original. It concerned itself with mechanisms whose instructions were modified by information received from the device executing the instructions (by feed-back). Publication of much of this work was delayed by security considerations, but when it saw the light of day it became generally apparent, as it had long been to those directly concerned with the original mathematical formulations, that the mathematics applied to automatic pilots and the like could serve in any situation in which control was exerted. The science, or super-science, of cybernetics was born.

Furthermore, any work done on the formation of control devices had to concern itself not only with the processing of information but with the nature of information itself. Once these problems had been solved, it was possible to build a mechanism that would process information in a manner determined by those who were currently programming it, such a flexible device being called a computer.

The situation of the engineers and mathematicians at this stage was almost precisely analogous to that of the physiologists of the first half of the twentieth century: the engineers had solved most of the problems of power and had come up against those of complex control equipment, much as Pavlov reached what he called the barrier of the brain. Furthermore, the valves and their linkages in early control devices were noted to be strikingly similar to the neurones and neuronal organization of the more elemental parts of the human brain, and some of the faults developing in ill-designed control mechanisms were found to be recognizable in human beings with gross neurological damage.

When the computer-engineers moved on to the production of large and immensely complicated computing machines they entered the realm of psychology as surely as their discoveries and accomplishments made cyberneticists of psychologists.

For in producing things that would take in information, consider or process it, and make an appropriate selection affected not only by recent information but past experience, they were making mechanisms that acted intelligently and therefore, to dismiss a controversy that was never more than terminological, possessed intelligence.

By concerning themselves with a general science of mechanism, not confined to devices already made but including the most complex computers and controllers conceivable, the engineers did calculations the wide applicability of which included the specialized computer array comprising the central nervous sytem. As the nineteen-sixties opened, the engineers also began to consolidate their practical knowledge of the mysteries and weaknesses of giant computers, and pointed out the dramatic possibilities of these mechanisms, over and above their ability to perform high-speed analyses of data. They showed that there was a theoretical limit to the degree of development of computers that could take place without breakdown – and pointed out that alone of the animals man, with his hypertrophied cerebrum, experienced functional psychoses. As an aside, to deal with objections to the imposition of mechanistic theories on mankind, they cited mathematical proof that a device was constructible that could reproduce itself, and that there was no reason why such a device should not be designed so that it could process information in the same way as man, show the same learning pattern and, if requested, be preprogrammed to lie convincingly about its phantasy-life.

The computers themselves, used as tools in experimental work, have catalysed an alteration in our views about what constitutes respectable scientific theory. The old idea that the scientific method consisted essentially of making a hypothesis on the basis of established facts, doing an experiment (preferably with only one variable) crucial for that hypothesis, and extending the hypothesis if experimental support were forthcoming until eventually a clear law, like those put forward by Newton, resulted, must be put on one side when very complex systems are being investigated. This is because a hypothesis can only be made if a sizeable proportion of the existing facts about a system is known (as it may be in cosmology but is not in psychology or other sciences of like scope, such as economics), and because the main function of a hypothesis, apart from producing a feeling of comfort, is pointing to which stimulus (or input) to vary in the subsequent experiment, which nowadays is not necessary; the computers, opening up to us immense possibilities of doing what would once have been endless calculations, enable us to allow everything to vary, the interrelationships of the parts being worked out later by multivariate analysis.

In psychological experiment it is virtually impossible to allow only one factor to vary and the extreme artificiality of such laboratories as enable us to arrange this, such as Pavlov's isolation-chambers for his dogs, means that if alternative computer-aided experimental opportunities exist for weighing the trends in organisms under more natural circumstances, they should be taken.

The corollary of all this is that we must forget, once and for all, the idea that somewhere, somehow, the answer will be found: there is no answer in the study of man's thinking, but a series of answers, all less precise than arithmetic though more reliable than wise sayings about the weather, and their sum will give us the basis of a sound probabilistic science. Even today, the public and many members of the profession still look for certainty of a level that can only be found in Newtonian science, and each new variant of research in psychiatry is scanned for signs that precise formulations may be forthcoming. The transfer of these hopes from Freudian psychology to social psychiatry, or from Pavlovian theory to Existentialist psychiatry is unjustified not because of the failure of the newer approaches but because the hopes themselves are misplaced.

Computer engineers and cyberneticists are inclined to make exuberant forecasts that within ten years a computer will be world chess champion; and that if the massive pre-programming required is undertaken and the public can be trained to put up with it, computers can usurp the doctor's diagnostic function. More soberly, they say that cybernetics, alone of the many contenders, provides a basis for a scientific psychiatry because no other method is able to deal with the enormous complexity of the central nervous system and its interactions with a constantly shifting environment.

I am not competent to assess these claims, but the practical and heuristic potential of computers and cybernetic concepts in psychology and psychiatry, as in so many other biological sciences, can hardly be overstated.

The Causation of
Schizophrenia

Schizophrenia and the affective illnesses (illnesses of mood) are the two major psychoses, dominating all other psychiatric illness: the commonest reason for long-term psychiatric hospitalization is schizophrenia and the commonest presenting symptom in psychiatry is depression. These psychoses have in common certain qualities that set them apart from the personality abnormalities and the reactions called psychoneuroses: the nature of the failure of function is more profound, the whole of the personality is involved, the reactions of the patient differ not only in degree but in kind from the way healthy people react, the illnesses go in families in a fashion that seems more clear-cut than with neurosis, the psychological precipitation of the illness may be trivial or impossible to find (or non-existent) and the illnesses occur only rarely before adolescence and more commonly at epochs of physiological imbalance such as the menopause.

As briefly mentioned earlier, *schizophrenia* consists of a series of associated failures of function which for the purposes of description and investigation are grouped under certain headings, but which overlap and intermingle in different patients and which may not all be present in an individual case.

The schizophrenic process produces a fragmentation of the different functional aspects of the mind, a disintegration that leads to strange, illogical, and disconnected thoughts and activities. The man who, having once been well and normal, develops acute schizophrenia will display disorder of thought, delusions and incongruity of emotional response, disorders of muscular movements and speech, and disintegration which, if untreated, gets progressively worse. Most patients with schizophrenia show most of these symptoms to some degree, and the type of schizophrenia (paranoid, catatonic, hebe-phrenic, or simple) is assessed according to the most prominent set of symptoms. The pictures seen in the acute illnesses can be fairly specific to these sub-types, but as described in the intro-ductory chapter the distinctions fade as the illness lasts longer than two years (i.e. becomes chronic), with the different symp-toms appearing less dramatically and usually some representa-tions of all of the main schizophrenic abnormalities appearing in roughly equal degree; so that commonly the sub-grouping is abandoned as time goes by and the patients are designated simply as 'chronic schizophrenics'. At this stage their main characteristics are likely to be those of oddity, social withdrawal, awkwardness of gait and speech, and a tendency, if the right questions are put, to air rather stereotyped and stale delusional ideas.

Schizophrenia is the most tragic state to be commonly found in the institutions of a civilized country. Its cause is unknown.

Ten years ago many psychiatrists would have wagered that by ten years from then the great puzzle would have been solved. Today some psychiatrists would say the same, and indeed a few would say that the answer has already been found. Certainly many feel that we have the information, that all that is needed is a masterly synthesis. But the more theories that exist, the less likely it is that any of them is the correct one, and at the present time no one theory explains all the observa-tions or carries predictive value.

Freudian psychoanalysts and psychotherapists of allied schools have sometimes seen in the schizophrenic patients they studied a kind of consistency, an internal logic, a residuum of normality, or some other attribute that led them to suppose that it should be possible, by psychotherapy more radical and more profound than that demanded by the psychoneuroses, to reintegrate the disintegrated minds of their patients. Some have supposed that the schizophrenic's withdrawal from stress at the moment of entering adult life could be interpreted as a gross regression to an infantile state of dependency, postulating, with psychological explanations that could be made to fit the picture only by a *tour de force*, a psychogenesis for the illness, a basis in childhood trauma (together with predisposition and, later, precipitating factors).

Viewed as specific therapy, psychoanalysis and related methods have proved failures in this illness, for the most helpful kind of therapy does not urge the patient to air his psychotic ideas but encourages him instead to put them to one side and to attend to the realities of the world, to social intercourse, to useful and gainful activity, and to life as it goes on round him. But any kind of individual attention to the schizophrenic patient has always been rewarding, and many of the *social* improvements now obtained must have arisen from the encouraging effects of making contact with the withdrawn and unresponsive patient that the initiators of this type of therapy were able to demonstrate.

All of the readers of this book must be interested to some extent in how their minds work. Many who study medicine do so because of an interest not only in their fellow-men but in themselves and their own peculiarities, and the same applies even more strongly to those who go on to study psychiatry. Curiosity about the workings of the body or mind can often be satisfied, as any general practitioner will agree, by a formula which is not in itself helpful, but which conveys the assurance that no mystery exists; so that a patient will be satisfied if he is told that his aching back is the consequence of lumbago (=aching back) or that his indigestion is caused by functional dyspepsia (=indigestion). Doctors also plump if they can for the simple explanation, and if it seems at first sight to explain the facts, may not care to examine it too closely lest it turn out false; the recent discoveries about diabetes, which make it obvious that the supposition that the illness depended solely on a reduction in the production of insulin is no longer valid, have elicited not only interest but a modicum of disappointment that an illness once thought to be fully worked out should now turn out once again to be a mystery.

In general medicine and the organically based psychological illnesses doctors are able to proceed along logical lines of investigation, shedding light on the darkness and making order out of chaos in a way that can be described in ordinary English (though jargon may be used to save time and preserve the professional image) and which respects the usual assumptions about cause and effect. Corresponding efforts in psychiatry often have to depend on the use of words as the tool for both investigation and the induction of laws, and though many of the phenomena of the psychoneuroses can be described and some of the steps in unconscious mental processes can be hinted at, the probability is that words and language are not adequate to describe a large proportion of the symptoms of schizophrenia (the schizophrenic, faced with this actual problem, may neologize, i.e. make up new words because none of the old ones will do) and are totally inadequate for accounting for the development of schizophrenic manifestations out of normal psychological events.

For example, one can perhaps imagine being a conscientious, over-clean, tense person; and then that a hideously unclean thought or temptation crosses the mind and is rejected, giving rise nevertheless to guilty anxiety; and that the anxiety, mingled with a sense of uncleanliness, forces one, like Pontius Pilate, to wash the hands: and that thus the germ of an obsessional neurosis, with compulsive hand-washing, is born.

But it is not so easy to see, no matter how hard one may try and how skilfully the verbal symbols may be juggled, how any form of stress or anxiety or insecurity, no matter how extreme or prolonged or complicated, could make one hear a voice saying, 'No, it isn't!' at the back of the head and an answering voice saying, 'Yes, it is!' at the front, or could make one *know* (not suspect, or be inclined to believe, but *know*) that one was a member of the Royal Family and the rightful heir to the Throne.

Nevertheless, the human temptation to look for and the need to postulate a verbally sequential chain of events in the genesis of schizophrenia is great, and it would be wrong to be put off simply because the task seems difficult. For my part, my working belief is that words are not suited to the purpose, and that attempts at using them in order to make clear the basic mechanisms of schizophrenia are foredoomed; but it is impossible not to admire the ingenuity and diligence of those who have worked on this subject in this way, and their descriptions of the psychology of schizophrenics and those in their milieu have added greatly to our appreciation of the psychological factors associated (as I would think, not necessarily causally) with schizophrenia.

The inquiring reader, in the face of conflicting theories and not in possession of enough evidence to be able to decide for himself, would probably best be served by having the results of a kind of consensus of present-day psychiatrists, in order that he could know at least which of the theories was the most popular and which the least. No such intra-professional survey has been done but I should hazard that most European psychiatrists would postulate that a constitutional fault leading to a bio-chemical imbalance is the likely nature of the pathology of the illness; that a sizeable minority believes that psychological factors – early environmental stress – fashion the disease; and that both factions respect the evidence that conflicts with their own favourite.

Before dealing with the biochemical theories of the illness, and the chemical abnormalities so far found, I think it advisable to describe and, in so far as I feel able, evaluate psychodynamic and other explanations of the predisposition of certain persons to this profound disease, asking the reader to remember that the biochemical and the psychodynamic explanations of schizo-phrenia do not really conflict; they may be describing the same processes in different terms or accounting for separate links in a long causal chain.

Most of the well-planned studies of psychodynamics and early environmental influences are being done in the U.S.A., where this type of comprehensive, time-consuming, and expensive work was pioneered. To illustrate the scope of some of the endeavours, at Yale not only may the patient receive intensive study, but the dynamics (i.e. the psychological trends and types of reaction) of all the members of his immediate family are individually determined and compared: one clinician admits to his wards not only the schizophrenic but the parents and any brothers or sisters who will come in as well, in order that family dynamics and interactions may be more precisely defined and

their importance determined. Our knowledge of the inter-
actions and roles of the members of a normal family being what
it is (not much), comprehensive long-term work on normals
might be more valuable at this stage, but a fascinating picture
of the state of affairs in the families of schizophrenics is painted
by these workers, among whom the teams of Lidz and Bateson
are perhaps the best known.

From the start the child who is destined to become schizophrenic in adult life has, it is said, an unusual and unsuitable
emotional environment. The schizophrenic's mother comes in
for most of the criticism, some of it extremely harsh: she is
characteristically described as possessive, subtly dominating,
manipulative, exploitive, distrustful, hostile, devious, rejecting,
combining strictness with over-concern about the child's sexual
behaviour, and liable to be more self-assured and dominating
than the father. Though unable to give spontaneous love, this
virago intrudes, allowing her child no privacy. The father's
fault is not so much that he has positive faults as that he fails to
counter-balance the aggregate of the mother's malignant
qualities. Interestingly enough the family pattern of dominating,
intrusive mother and passive father is more frequently found
among lower-class families, where it may be said to be a normal
variant; and the lower social classes have, in fact, a higher risk
of schizophrenia than the upper classes.

In this family situation the child is further prevented from
normal development by ambiguities in the relationships between
the parents and between himself and his parents. Usually overt
distrust exists between members of the family or, if it does not,
something called 'pseudomutuality', a kind of masked distrust,
looking to a casual observer like trust, is present instead. In
either case the subject's interpretations of his environment
naturally become less consistent and therefore, the theory goes,
easier to relinquish should illness supervene.

The child has difficulty in deciding his role within the family
and thus his social development is further retarded. Most of all,
our sympathy is demanded by the ordeal called the 'double-
bind'. This requires for its existence an intense emotional
relationship between two people, and the passing of two types

of message simultaneously from one person to the other, the situation being such that the recipient of the messages cannot clarify or comment on the disparity he notes. An example of this type of communication or non-communication would be a mother saying to her young son, 'Come here, darling,' in a tone that boded ill for him when he got there. If the son demurs, he must explain why, and the mother may and probably will deny that there was any threat in her tone; if the boy goes to his mother he must ignore a message, the unspoken one, in which he puts great faith. He therefore remains irresolute, seeking further data but unable to obtain it by the normal means of communication. The mother may go on to ask, 'What's the matter? You're not afraid of your mother, are you?' If the boy has been awaiting a solution, he is disappointed, for he is merely confirmed in the double-bind: he is afraid, of course, but he cannot answer Yes because little boys are not afraid of their mummies, who love them; he cannot answer No, not only because he is afraid, but because he would then have to prove he wasn't by going to her. This double-bind situation, multiplied many times over and repeated by the parents in their reactions one with the other, makes the child mistrust the sensory data he perceives.

It is postulated that all this, and no doubt other confusions still undescribed, make the child have a compelling need to withdraw, so that when the child becomes adolescent and then enters early adult life, with a plethora of social, emotional, and intellectual problems clamouring to be solved by means which the subject deeply mistrusts and cannot skilfully manipulate, he abandons reality and becomes frankly schizophrenic. One psychiatrist jibs at proposing that these environmental factors can lead to schizophrenia directly, but suggests that the child so raised will prove an even more unsuitable parent, producing a more severe response in his own children, which in turn is magnified in the third generation and at this point becomes liable to lead to schizophrenia.

The formulations summarized above have, at least in the original, a near-poetic quality. It is easy to feel great sympathy for the child and to see how the child might want to escape from the life-trap, by no matter what method. That psychotherapy, the treatment that should work if the theory is right, does not in fact alter the outlook, does not disprove the hypothesis: it may well be that the child, like other young mammals, has critical periods for 'imprinting' certain skills and attitudes, so that, once lost, the opportunity for gaining trust and security is gone for ever. There are, however, other criticisms of these accounts of the childhoods of adult schizophrenics that carry considerable weight, and they may be used to counterbalance most of the arguments and interpretations just set out.

It is true, to take the first point first, that the mother of the schizophrenic is often a challenging specimen – cold, detached, and forceful; the father, too, may be odd and is often the non-dominant partner. But this is not always the case: the working psychiatrist can think of dozens of sets of parents of schizophrenics who were, or seemed, perfectly normal and whose homes were or seemed repositories of trust. To argue, as some ardent dynamicists will, that the apparent normality of the parents is phoney and that what passes for trust is 'pseudo-mutuality' is to say not only that things are often not what they seem, which is acceptable, but that how things seem is not the best guide to what they are, a way of thinking that, to enter into the spirit of the argument, is only excusable in those who have themselves had too intensive a course of double-binds.

The patient's relationship with his parents is determined, in the retrospective studies (i.e. those done after the patient has presented as a schizophrenic), by asking a schizophrenic about the past, or by asking disturbed or worried parents about the past, or by determining the family dynamics by observing them after a member of the family has fallen seriously ill. It might be predicted that abnormalities would be found, even if all that you could say with confidence would be that the parents would be at once self-reproachful and on the defensive.

But what constitutes an abnormality in family life and what does not is a study in itself, and one that has not yet been done, so that in the same way that physiognomies may look odd when we go abroad, because for once we look at them instead of through them, family relationships may look odd in the schizophrenic's family because we have studied no others in comparable detail, and because the subjects alter self-consciously under scrutiny. Much of the attraction of the double-bind hypothesis, to underline the argument, lies not in its oddity, which would be congruous with its role in the production of a singularly odd illness, but in its familiarity. We know about it because we have all experienced it, but few of us are schizophrenic.

The explanation of the coolness and distance of the mother and father, and the poor relationship with the child, may spring from the nature of the personalities of patients destined to become schizophrenic and those of their close relatives, for the personality most closely associated genetically and premonitorily with schizophrenia is cool, distant, and poor at social contacts and emotional intercourse. When neither parent possesses this type of personality, but by some chance confluence of genes the child does, the ambiguities and hidden hostilities noted in the parent–child relationships may arise from the inability of the parents to get the emotional contact and rapport with this child that they had with their others. And if the family difficulties do, in fact, lead to schizophrenia, though non-specific as far as current analyses can determine, why do they not also lead to behaviour disorder – to tantrums, or rebellion, or despair? They do not, for the rare controlled study shows no distinguishing features between the childhoods of those who become schizophrenic and those who remain healthy.

Less criticism can be made of the theoretical constructions of those psychotherapists who study and treat the condition of *childhood schizophrenia*. Despite the verbal coincidence, some would say that childhood schizophrenia, though it possesses certain features in common with adult schizophrenia and has, if anything, an even worse prognosis, is a different illness, with, correspondingly, a different constitutional and psychological basis; it is convenient, nevertheless, to discuss the illness at this point, with the psychodynamic features of schizophrenics' families freshly in mind.

Childhood schizophrenia is a strange aberration, consisting

of many variable features, but with evidence of chaotic motor activity, inability to express or deal with emotion in any appropriate way, inability to satisfy instinctive desires, the performance in many cases of meaningless but tenaciously retained rituals, social withdrawal of a peculiar kind, and a mixture of inability to learn and the development of islands of normal or supernormal skill. As may be supposed the complex function of speech is usually severely affected. Untreated, the outlook is almost hopeless: fortunately the disease is rare.

Psychotherapists approach the illness through consideration of the patient's psychodynamics because they have to: none of the physical treatments that have coincided with the spectacular changes in expectation of cure in adult schizophrenia have produced similar benefits among the children. But their work is so arduous and expensive in time that they more than most hope that other treatments will arise that will render theirs obsolete.

In general the schizophrenic child has, quite apart from his later psychological stress, had a hard time of it from the moment he prepared himself for the birth-trauma. Not only is he likely to have a genetic loading of schizophrenic relatives, but the circumstances of his birth and his post-natal period are likely to have been more bedevilled by organic illness than most.

It is his psychological environment that has been so exhaustively studied, however, as the main avenue of therapeutic hope. It is said that the children become ill because of 'conflictual' living: critical external strain coincides with or reinforces critical internal strain in the home at the outset of the illness in many of the case-histories. The normal child, leaving his mother's side at about the age of eighteen months, indulges in repetitive play and ritualistic activity as if seeking uniformity; the schizophrenic child, one theorist says, does this also, but to excess. It may be that inability to accomplish the parting and indulge in exploratory and coordinating activity accounts for the uncertainty that schizophrenic children have about the boundaries of their bodies (the body-image), which are mapped out over this period in the normal course of events.

The child seems to develop wishes for basic sensual pleasures like cuddling that are in some way warped and are treated by the child as threatening, so that the child feels that they are too hazardous to indulge and deals with them by withdrawal.

Arguments against this formulation of the causation of schizophrenia echo those adduced against the psychodynamic theory of adult schizophrenia. The mother's point of view is usually that the initial failure was one of response in the child; and this, persisting, leads the mother to adopt varying types of approach in an attempt to make contact, a technique that is easy to label inconsistent (and therefore traumatic) when it is really the variable manifestation of a consistent desire for rapport.

Nevertheless, the psychodynamically oriented theorists have some heavy ammunition to support their approach to this illness. It is generally agreed in medicine that demonstration that a therapy is effective is not proof of the theory underlying its use. It is, all the same, persuasive, for the proof of the pudding must lie somewhere, and the fact is that at the Langley Porter Neuropsychiatric Institute in San Francisco the psychotherapists, after prodigal expenditure of time, money, and skill, and amid admissions that they would welcome fervently a specific drug for the illness, produce major improvement in about 20 per cent of the children they see, better figures than those from any source of comparable reliability, and proof, if more were needed, of their extraordinary optimism and skill.

In the introduction to this book *sociological studies* were described and some of the typical results given. Epidemiological and allied work is having a renaissance, and at present many of the chairs of psychiatry are occupied by physicians whose bent is towards field-study rather than the bedside.

Only the most enthusiastic seriously propose that sociological factors occupy the highest place on the list of causal factors in (the undoubtedly multiple causation of) schizophrenia, but the success of altering the style of mental hospitals, described in Chapter 5, leaves us in no doubt as to the importance of social factors in the treatment of the established illness. These factors will emerge in a later section, then, and apart from saying that the general proposal is that the predisposed person or the schizophrenic in temporary remission is more likely to develop or redevelop the symptoms of the illness in circumstances of social isolation, the sociological arguments will not be elaborated at this point. Sociological studies are becoming more useful in psychiatry as they take in finer and finer detail, and it is significant that psychopathological studies by post-Freudian theorists have most usefully expanded in the direction of examining social factors; the two disciplines are likely to meet, to their mutual benefit.

An interesting theory of the basis of schizophrenia is the proposition that the illness is really a *perceptual abnormality*, that is that the schizophrenic acts oddly because the sensory data-processing equipment he possesses is faulty, in the same way that an aircraft landing automatically in fog would fly erratically if its mechanism misinterpreted the information received from the ground. Such an explanation is really only another way of stating the problem, but no restatement is beneath our notice at the present stage of knowledge. This aspect of schizophrenia has gained in interest from its connexion with experiments done on sensory deprivation as a prelude to launching astronauts.

The person who is floated in warm still water wearing a black opaque mask through which he breathes, or who is otherwise deprived of the usual nervous impulses we get from sense organs scanning the outside world, undergoes some very odd experiences. He loses temporarily some of his ability to learn and memorize, and becomes for a time less able to maintain the 'constancies' (i.e. to judge that a man in the middle distance is the same size as a man in the foreground despite the different heights of the images they throw on the observer's retina); he may also find three-dimensional vision difficult to achieve again after the experiment. Most dramatic of all, the sense-deprived normal subject may undergo hallucinatory experiences, mostly visual and mostly apparently dependent for their inception on a modicum of light penetrating the apparatus, but all increasing as the duration of the deprivation periods extends.

This type of experience has something in common with a schizophrenic episode; schizophrenics tend to see the world as a two-dimensional affair (this tendency being measurable by psychological tests); constancy of perception also breaks down, the schizophrenic being unable to take into account the distance of the perceived object when assessing its size, and unaided by clues which three-dimensional perception would provide. He is also likely, of course, to be hallucinated.

The obvious way to test the proposition that most readily arises – that sense-deprivation of a subtle kind is at the back of schizophrenic symptoms – is to subject schizophrenic subjects to full sense-deprivation in the expectation that they will tolerate it badly and that their perceptual and hallucinatory symptoms will get worse. This has been done, but in the event the schizophrenics did not alter for the worse: if anything, their hallucinations lessened, and they tolerated the unpleasant aspects of the experiment better than most normal subjects, as they weather most forms of discomfort better than the rest of us.

The current research on sense-deprivation is being done, in the light of the negative results with schizophrenia, at a neurological rather than a psychiatric level, but it remains an important technical advance in the study of perception.

Perceptual disorders in the schizophrenic cover more fields than size-constancy and three-dimensionality; the 'existentialist' psychiatrists, interesting themselves in understanding and analysing the phenomena experienced by the schizophrenic patient, describe anomalies of perception not only of space but of time, while experimental work confirms that the schizophrenic gauges time-intervals differently from the normal subject. In the field of psychological testing the schizophrenic displays other anomalies such as 'over-inclusion', i.e. an inclination to see the trees, the sky, and the fields around rather than simply the wood, but though this may be illustrated by giving perceptual examples it is probably a general characteristic of the kind of thinking that goes with the schizophrenic process.

There are still some pathologists who aver that schizophrenia is an *organic disease*, meaning that abnormalities of structure can be demonstrated in the central nervous system post-mortem. The biochemical theories refer to errors of function rather than of structure, but their popularity depends largely on the feeling among some psychiatrists that schizophrenia has much in common with the organic types of reaction seen in intoxications and after brain damage. In Germany, K. Kleist tried to produce a scheme of schizophrenia that was linked with cortical function, making his formulation a purely neurological one relying on outdated concepts of localization of function in the cortex. Many of his clinical descriptions and pointers for the prediction of a patient's outlook were excellent, but his work has not gained acceptance. All the same, even such schizophrenic features as failure of perceptual mechanisms are seen in the brain-damaged subject, and pathologists still continue to look for, and from time to time report prematurely that they have found, microscopic abnormalities in the brains of deceased schizophrenics.

Biochemical aspects of schizophrenia have been studied for many years, and each discovery of some abnormality of metabolism, of blood-chemistry, or of constituents of the urine has seemed to promise fresh strides and has, as like as not, engendered some exuberant theory. The possibility of a toxin being responsible for schizophrenia has been in psychiatric minds for more than a century; Kraepelin himself suggested at the end of the nineteenth century that 'auto-intoxication' might be a cause.

However, until a decade or so ago the biochemical investigations done on schizophrenics were mostly negative or the results spurious. Only Gjessing, working in Norway, using detailed methods and techniques, managed to do work of lasting value and to set the correct style for later investigators. He was aware that simply working with schizophrenic patients and looking for abnormalities which the group had in common was the wrong way to go about it, for, as he said, it was far from certain that patients with schizophrenia constituted a homogeneous group; they might really be a group of patients who had different diagnoses (and, therefore, chemistries) though roughly similar outward appearances; and it is worth remembering, in this context, that Bleuler, who coined the name schizophrenia, actually used the plural, describing the schizophrenias. Gjessing preferred, in the absence of any data from which a start could be made, to find a small group of schizophrenics with illnesses so sharply defined by their symptoms and course that it was highly likely that they were all of a kind, and to study their metabolism intensively. He settled on the group called Periodic Catatonics, patients who develop recurrent catatonic schizophrenic illnesses and have intervening periods of normality or near-normality. Their periods of near-normality gave him the chance to determine normal base-lines for his various measurements and assays, and during periods of catatonia the procedure could be repeated.

His care and foresight were repaid by unequivocal results. He showed that the nitrogen metabolism (principally protein breakdown and build-up) followed a phasic course that matched the catatonic symptoms so that, once the relationship between the nitrogen-phase and the catatonia-phase could be determined for an individual patient (this being variable), the onset of catatonic symptoms could be predicted. Not only that, but, nitrogen metabolism being alterable by administration of thyroid hormone, he was able to control the phasic tendency of his catatonics' metabolism and thus prevent the recurrence of overt catatonic schizophrenia. This work, done largely before the Second World War and refined and confirmed since that time, remains a model for present-day investigators. In itself, however, it led to a therapeutic brick wall, because thyroid hormone was ineffective in other types of schizophrenia, and other schizophrenics do not show alterations of nitrogen metabolism of this kind, while the illness called periodic catatonia is rare, so that no great inroads were made on the size of the mental hospital population following the publication of this work.

Some of the difficulties inherent in determining *essential* differences between the body-fluids (plasma, serum, urine, etc.) of schizophrenics and those of normals can be gauged by remarking some of the *inessential* differences between the schizophrenic patient and the normal person: the schizophrenic is likely to be in hospital, while the normal is freer and more active; the patient may not be able to afford many cigarettes and will not drink alcohol, while the normal pleases himself; the diets differ, that of the patient being, unhappily, monotonous and cheap and that of the normal person variable but in general better; and so on. At the level of subtlety of the chemical changes reported in the literature, these differences in mode of life can account for the whole of the set of differences noted in an experiment. Thus, in order that these variations may be minimized it is necessary to have both schizophrenics and controls (I shall use this term for normal subjects used for comparison with patients) matched for age, living in the same area, under the same régimes of exercise, eating the same diets, and allowed the same luxuries; it would also be helpful if their emotions could be kept approximately even, but this is not easy to arrange. The rest of it, however, is being done, and as might be expected from its scope, it is being done best in the United States.

The results of strictly chemical investigations may be summarized fairly briefly. Apart from Gjessing's work nothing done before about 1950 holds much water, though the schizophrenic's apparent ability to tolerate enormous dosages of insulin, remarked during insulin-coma therapy, remains unexplained.

More recently it has been found that a substance called *ceruloplasmin*, which is an alpha-globulin associated with the carrying of copper in a bound form in the blood, is increased in acute schizophrenia; it increases in other illnesses too, however, and it may be that, like the high counts of white blood cells seen in a variety of acute illnesses, the ceruloplasmin increase is part of a compensatory or defence process. Interest in ceruloplasmin has lessened since its variability with diet (particularly vitamins) and with emotions was discovered, but it is linked with a comprehensive theory of the chemical cause of psychosis and will be mentioned again later.

Another substance called *taraxein*, a qualitatively different form of ceruloplasmin, is said not only to be present in greater quantities in schizophrenic blood, but to be capable of producing psychotic symptoms if injected into a normal person: the validity of this work is uncertain at the time of writing, though the experimental design was admirable and the observations were made under what is called double-blind (see p. 82) conditions.

A technique called chromatography has recently been used to

investigate body fluids. It enables different substances to be separated out in a way that would be impossible or almost so by orthodox chemical methods. Various differences found in schizophrenics' urines have turned out to be the consequences of such non-schizophrenic foibles as a liking for coffee, but with better-controlled studies substances such as indoles have been extracted from the urine which hold out some promise in that they may themselves be used for biological experiment, i.e. in the determination of their effect on animal behaviour and on behaviour and consciousness in man.

Determination of the toxic effects of schizophrenic body fluids, then, provides another avenue of advance. It has long been known that schizophrenic body fluids were more toxic than those of the normal, but only recently have the variables of abode and diet been satisfactorily controlled. The fluids have been injected into a variety of experimental animals, from men down to fighting fish, and some of the effects are striking and possibly significant.

In the laboratory the effects of body-fluids on enzymes (organic catalysts derived from cells) may be determined, but this test-tube work, though more accurate and objective and thus in a way more satisfying than that done on living organisms, has so far come to nothing.

Animal work consists essentially of the injection of some extract from a schizophrenic into the animal, followed by observations of the effect, particularly the effect on motor activity (seeking catatonic symptoms). There have been some apparently positive results. One substance obtained from schizophrenic urine produced catatonic symptoms in the experimental animal and periods of exaltation have been described (the animal workers have or seem to have extraordinary insight into the moods of their charges). More complex observations have been done on rats trained to climb a vertical rope, the standard time for the climb being known; after the administration of plasma from psychotic patients the rats became not only slower but odd and peculiar in their actions, sometimes pausing and staring dreamily into space.

The most striking experiments have been done on a large

and impressive spider, appropriately named Zilla X. Notata. This animal builds symmetrical and beautiful webs in a stereotyped but meaningful way when well, and its web remains at the end of a period of activity as objective evidence of its levels of functioning. Certain spiders were fed with a sac containing schizophrenic serum and coated with sugar, and their web-building after they imbibed the contents was compared with that of controls. The serum from patients suffering from most forms of schizophrenia produced no change in web-building activity; that from catatonic schizophrenics, however, was associated with a significant reduction in webs built and those that were done were rudimentary in form.

In experiments on man, the results are so far doubtful. Understandably, early work consisted of giving normal serum to schizophrenics and observing the results, rather than the other way round, and some transient successes were reported, but the experiments, though bold, were not designed in such a way that the results can be relied upon. It is necessary always to remember that in psychiatry any procedure, no matter how purposeless, is likely to produce some improvement simply because, in carrying it out, contact is made with the patient and he becomes the centre of interest and attention. More recently extracts of schizophrenic serum have been administered to normal subjects, some of them prison volunteers, and transient schizophrenic-like symptoms resulted; the Tulane group, giving taraxein, obtain the most clear-cut symptoms.

A group of Russian psychiatrists, working from Kraepelin's hypothesis that some of the schizophrenics' illnesses might be due to toxin from the body's metabolism or from outside, have approached the matter from a different standpoint. In Russia psychiatrists, in common with their other medical colleagues, have provided a welcome buffer between the state and the people, but they sometimes appear, in their over-evaluation of the excellent work of Pavlov, to be compensating for their frequent moments of independence by clinging to a safe orthodoxy undesirable in those concerned with the development of a young science.

Criticisms on grounds of dogmatism would not be confined

to psychiatrists from the communist countries, however, and certainly the Russian psychiatrists' approach to the theory of the schizophrenic toxin was not notable for its orthodoxy. They proposed, simply, that if the toxin came from outside it most probably came from food, and if it came from inside it must come from the breakdown of food or food products, so the best thing to do would be to try starvation. Put in this way, it sounds as though their idea was merely a variant of the iniquitous practices of bleeding and debilitation carried out in the notorious Hoxton madhouses of the nineteenth century, but no one seeing the psychiatrists concerned in the trial working with their patients could entertain such an analogy.

The patients and their relatives were first asked if they agreed to the therapy, and if permission was forthcoming all drugs were stopped and then starvation was started: the patients felt hungry for forty-eight hours or so, and then the feeling of hunger left them. They subsisted on fizzy drinks and vitamins after that and continued normal activities; at the end of three weeks or so hunger returned and constituted a signal for starting feeding the patients again. In the absence of controls, of adequate numbers, and of other requirements ignored by the Russians, it is not easy to evaluate the striking and sometimes dramatic improvements that consistently resulted; as a later chapter (Chapter 2) will make clear, the easiest results to obtain in any therapeutic trial are misleadingly optimistic ones. But properly planned and controlled experiments producing the same results would be a powerful argument in favour of the organic theory of causation of schizophrenia, quite apart from being therapeutically beneficial.

The most plausible comprehensive *biochemical theory of schizophrenic causation* is that associated with the names of Osmond and Smythies and later of Hoffer, which links the drugs such as mescaline and lysergic acid (L.S.D.) that are called hallucinogens, and the normally occurring substance called adrenaline.

The drug *mescaline*, an alkaloid found in mescal, obtained from the dumpling cactus, produces abnormal and bizarre psychic and perceptual effects. Among other manifestations of mescaline intoxication, which has been widely described by laymen since the turn of the century and which had a vogue recently in the Western hemisphere, are unusual and inappropriate emotions, derealization (a sense of being cut off or detached), disorders of body-image, of time and space perception and of vision, hallucinations (largely visual), and the ascription of significance to unimportant stimuli (ideas of reference). Thus the mescaline psychosis resembles the schizophrenic psychosis more closely than any other intoxication.

The substance *adrenaline* is, as is well known, concerned in the reactions to threatening stimuli, and it produces many of the outward and inward signs of anxiety, fear, and rage. It, or a close analogue, has another function, that of transmitting the nerve impulse across the synapse (junction) between certain nerves. It is thought from its distribution and other evidence that it is one of the agents performing this function in the central nervous system, though the synaptic mechanisms in the brain are not known in any detail.

In 1950 Osmond and Smythies remarked on the resemblance between the configuration of the mescaline molecule and that of the adrenaline molecule, and they proposed in effect that the symptoms of schizophrenia, especially acute and dramatic (often called 'florid') schizophrenia, might be the consequence of intoxication with some abnormal breakdown product (metabolite) of adrenaline, or some normal breakdown product in abnormal quantities. Few of the metabolites of adrenaline were known, but they suggested that *adrenochrome* (a bright-reddish coloured substance) might be suitable for study. Osmond went to Saskatchewan, and there, with Hoffer, continued to consider the hypothesis and to plan and perform experiments. Soon evidence appeared to support the theory: an asthmatic reported a lingering episode of mental peculiarity after using in his spray adrenaline that had gone pink through deterioration: adrenochrome produced a 'model' psychosis in those who tried it out, and adrenolutin, a further breakdown product of adrenochrome, was implicated in the pathology.

The final proposal was that adrenaline broke down to adrenochrome and that further breakdown was either to

5,6-dihydroxy-N-methylindole, which did not matter, or to adrenolutin, which might matter if it was produced to excess, since it could produce or combine in producing the schizophrenic's symptoms. Large quantities of adrenolutin might be produced if an individual preferentially broke down his adrenaline in that manner, or if the production and subsequent breakdown of abnormal amounts of adrenaline forced the level of adrenolutin up (as might happen, for example, as a consequence of the psychological stress and anxiety some researchers think important in the precipitation of schizophrenia).

Ceruloplasmin, the copper-binding alpha-globulin mentioned earlier in this section, and taraxein, also briefly mentioned, were tied in by explaining that ceruloplasmin bound adrenolutin irreversibly (i.e. combined firmly with it, thus removing it from action: it will be remembered that ceruloplasmin is increased in acute schizophrenia and that this was thought possibly to be a defence mechanism), while taraxein (thought possibly to cause schizophrenic symptoms, not necessarily directly) displaced adrenolutin on the ceruloplasmin molecule, thus preventing the ceruloplasmin from protectively mopping up the excess of toxic adrenolutin.

Even if all this turned out to be true, it would still leave us a long way from basing any therapy on the hypothesis (not that this is in itself a criticism): for antidotes to the hallucinogens (as drugs such as mescaline are called) do not benefit acute schizophrenics. The main criticisms of the theory are not so utilitarian, however: dissenters usually start off by pointing out that the mescaline psychosis, though it has some points of similarity with schizophrenia and is certainly more like schizophrenia than, say, being drunk, is still not very much like it. It does not involve the characteristic emotional flattening of schizophrenia – the subject is not only often emotionally enlivened but he may be guilt-stricken at the trouble he is causing those who are looking after him during his model psychosis, and deeply grateful for the sensations it is their kindness to provide; and it does not involve loss of insight – the mescaline-intoxicated subject says 'I am hallucinated' while the schizophrenic, in the unlikely event that he is visually hallucinated, may say 'Look at that!' expecting those around him to share his perceptions. Furthermore the administration of an hallucinogenic drug such as L.S.D. to a schizophrenic does not lead to a worsening of the schizophrenia; on the contrary, schizophrenics tolerate L.S.D. better than normals. Perhaps the principal feeling expressed about the theory is that it is premature, and that it is bolstered more by the liveliness of its presentation than the solidity of the experimental facts.

One of the most promising lines of research is linked with virology; the viruses are the smallest of the infective agents, smaller than bacteria and probably consisting of single large protein molecules. These viruses cause a wide range of illness from serious plagues like smallpox and poliomyelitis down to minor infections such as the common cold. After some virus illnesses the patient shows lassitude and a loss of well-being that is out of proportion to the severity of the illness itself. Some patients become severely depressed after influenza-like illnesses. It is conjectured that schizophrenia or some types of schizophrenia may be the sequels of infection with certain viruses, but the nature of the viruses concerned, if any, remains uncertain.

The more that psychiatrists and workers in allied fields pursue the will-o'-the-wisp of the causation of schizophrenia, the more distant it seems to become. The close study of the various aspects of the illness from angles determined by the scientific disciplines of those involved produces enormous quantities of information about the disease, and many factors can be correlated significantly with the presence of the illness; but in no case can it be said with certainty whether the factor correlated is cause or effect.

Our task would be easier if we knew what aspects to concentrate upon. As it is we hardly know where to start, and when the causation is discovered many psychiatrists alive today will find that they have spent their research time on wild-goose chases. There are compensations for this wasteful effort, for the researchers so far have disclosed ignorance of which they were hardly aware, largely of the range and quality of what we call normality; and this ignorance is now being remedied; also, it is a truism in psychiatry that causation is always multiple, which is to say that one seeks not the cause but the causes. A man who becomes anxious when his wife is pregnant and who develops a full-blown anxiety-state as the confinement expected in March approaches, may do so for a certain important reason but will rarely do so for that reason alone: the psychological causation may be that his mother died in childbirth when he was five and that this trauma reinforces the anxiety natural in the circumstances. But a physical cause, such as a series of heavy flu-like colds with complicating bronchitis, may also be a factor in reducing his resistance; and he may have a constitutional predisposition in that he has always been prone to anxiety, is usually nearer to an anxiety-state than most of the population, and has always been retiring and without close friends to take his troubles to.

Thus the triumphant production of the childhood bereavement as the 'cause' of the neurosis would be reckoned by a psychiatrist's colleagues not as perceptive but as jejune: the most you could say for it is that it might stand high on the list of causes when these are given ranks in the diagnostic formulation, and the least you could say for it would be that it is too late to do anything about it, whereas you can give antibiotics for the dull, obvious, but debilitating bronchitis. The fact, then, that the researches on schizophrenia have not elucidated the main cause does not mean that the work is wasted if auxiliary factors in the production or prolongation of the symptoms are disclosed; the 'cause', when it is found, may prove impossible to affect, in which case we must rely for logical treatment, as we rely now, on dealing with the auxiliary factors as best we can, a policy that produces good results despite its inelegance, as will be described in a later chapter (Chapter 5).

The directions the efforts take are decided largely by what techniques are available and by hints thrown out by therapeutic successes of various kinds. In medicine many problems are solved not solely by the application of the scientific method but by the focusing of it on a particular area or system. Pernicious anaemia was both fatal and mysterious until it was found that undercooked liver produced a total return to normality if taken regularly; once the pathologists and the biochemists knew of this effective treatment, they knew roughly where to look, and soon worked out what to look for. When some specific treatment for the schizophrenias is found, the end must be in sight. Until then, any new technique of investigation, whether it be chemical, psychological, psychometric, or any other, will be pressed into service on the off-chance that some good may come of it.

New Drugs in Psychiatry

2

Drugs used in psychiatry for the control of symptoms or the eradication of diseases are now so many and diverse that any general account of their development must be selective and, in this instance, influenced by the therapeutic usefulness of the products rather than their purely pharmacological, chemical, or structural interest. These drugs, many of which will be familiar to the reader from enthusiastic journalistic descriptions, may be divided at the outset into two main groups – those which are useful in treating schizophrenic psychoses, notably the pheno-thiazine drugs such as chlorpromazine (Largactil); and those used to elevate the mood, the anti-depressive drugs.

The *anti-schizophrenic* drugs, which are commonly though unhappily known as 'tranquillizers', are derived from two main sources: one large family stems from the substance pheno-thiazine, while two or three drugs of which the best known is reserpine (Serpasil) come from *Rauwolfia serpentina*, a climbing shrub found in India, or from closely related plants.

Phenothiazine itself, a molecule consisting essentially of two benzene rings linked by sulphur and nitrogen, was first used in veterinary practice, where it was extensively employed in the treatment of worms. It next received serious scrutiny after the start of the last war: in 1941, when the Japanese occupied the main sources of the anti-malarial drug, quinine, and when mepacrine (the synthetic drug developed in Germany by I. G. Farben and hastily manufactured in the United States) proved rather toxic and not completely effective, a vast cooperative research programme was undertaken to synthesize, examine, and test many compounds for suppressive anti-malarial properties. Among these compounds one or two derivatives of phenothiazine, which was already known from animal work to have some usefulness in ridding hosts of their parasites, were included. Though they proved ineffective it was later noted that they bore some resemblance to drugs being investigated in France for a different purpose, the anti-histamines.

The French workers at the Rhône–Poulenc laboratories started a comprehensive study of the pharmacology of these compounds, in which interest had lapsed in the United States. Compounds with various side-chains attached to the central phenothiazine nucleus were systematically assessed and soon some promising results were achieved. Anti-histamines such as promethazine (*Phenergan*), stronger than any previously produced, were made available for therapeutic use in the treatment of allergic conditions. The sedative actions of (Phenergan) made the drug unsuitable for use by patients who had to drive or perform skilled tasks; far from being regarded as a drawback, these sedative effects were exploited by French clinicians who used the drug as an aid in anaesthesia.

It was in an attempt to find a drug more suitable for anaesthetic and shock-preventing purposes that the systematic study of these phenothiazine compounds was extended. Many of the new substances were of great interest and pharmacological novelty, but it was not until a different series of analogues with a longer side-chain was elaborated that the most outstanding and, for psychiatry, the crucial compound, *chlorpromazine*, resulted.

When the central sedative effects of chlorpromazine were assessed they were found to be more striking than those of promethazine, but the drug also manifested an impressively large number of other actions (hence, by elision, the trade-name of Largactil), including anti-adrenaline, temperature-reducing, and nausea-preventing activity, and the capacity (called potentiation) of prolonging and increasing the activity of unrelated drugs given simultaneously for sedative or pain-killing purposes.

With so many actions chlorpromazine had obvious applications in many separate fields; even in the early nineteen-fifties, however, the possibility of using the drug to assist in the sedation of agitated psychiatric patients was one of the first to be explored. In those days the over-active, excited, or destructive patient could pose an almost insoluble problem in therapeutics; sedation, with orthodox drugs, of a degree great enough to produce freedom from agitation or combativeness was often achieved only at the cost of dangerous unsteadiness of gait or toxic side-effects and it was frequently found necessary to resort to the injection of morphine or the use of padded rooms or even, in countries where these measures were countenanced, of physical restraint.

The use of chlorpromazine to potentiate the sedatives already in use was attended by great improvement in the patients treated; indeed the effects were so far in excess of expectation that Delay and his associates suggested that the drug be tried on its own in psychiatric patients. In 1954 the first dramatic reports of its effectiveness started to appear in the psychiatric journals, and from that time on the drug took its place with sulphonamides and penicillin as one of the great chemotherapeutic agents of the twentieth century. No other drug has been investigated and written about in such detail, and few can have been prescribed in such quantities for so many patients, for apart from its powers of potentiation and its capacity to calm without producing clouding of consciousness, chlorpromazine appeared able, in a manner that is still not understood, to relieve specifically the symptoms of acute schizophrenia.

Because of its wide range of action the clear definition of how chlorpromazine could best be applied took several years of investigation, during which many of the patients who received the drug had it prescribed solely because of its tranquillizing effect. Correspondingly, the majority of such patients who were not in hospitals or institutions were psychoneurotic and complained principally of tension or anxiety, so that this anxiety-reducing effect was soon the best known to the press and public, and the generic term 'tranquillizer', already being popularized by other developments in the field of psychopharmacology, extended naturally to include chlorpromazine and subsequent similar drugs.

Psychiatrists, aware of the disparity between different drugs in this artificially grouped collection, struggled against using the word, but despite proposed substitute expressions like ataractic drugs and psychotropic drugs (themselves expressions with little to commend them), the term 'tranquillizer' seems to have prevailed.

As far as chlorpromazine is concerned, the paradoxical aspect of the term lies in the ultimate indications[1] that clinical researchers were able to define for the drug: it is now seldom used to render agitated or anxious neurotics tranquil, because of its depressing effect; and when it is successfully used in schizophrenia it removes whatever symptoms of the illness exist, so that if these include over-activity it may be said to tranquillize, while if they include, as they well may, under-activity and inertness, it activates. The nomenclature is thus not only inelegant but inaccurate and confusing; but it is established, and it is now customary in many centres to refer to the drugs effective in the schizophrenias as 'major tranquillizers' and the drugs effective in the eradication of psychoneurotic (exaggerated normal) anxiety as 'minor tranquillizers'.

The effects of chlorpromazine were more far-reaching than any study of the drug's pharmacology could have predicted. In the early nineteen-fifties the long-stay patients in most mental hospitals were far from ideally managed. Though the principles of occupation and retraining were well known, the salutary effects of humanitarian and individual treatment well documented, and the psychiatric and nursing staff well trained, inertia had come over the hospitals, and little difference between the ward-routine of those years and the routine of a decade or two before can now be discerned. Acutely ill patients were treated vigorously and, as far as knowledge permitted, well, but the chronically affected patients in the back wards of most hospitals lived a lost and formless life.

The use of occasional electrical treatment allowed some long-stay patients to be kept at a moderately good level of mental health, while others gained incidental advantage from the work-therapy aspect of helping in the ward kitchen or hospital

1. In the medical context the word *indication* refers to the symptoms or groups of symptoms which have been shown to respond to the treatment concerned, their presence thus indicating the therapy.

workshop; but in many refractory wards, despite the some-times over-enthusiastic use of leucotomy (see Chapter 4) to reduce the patients' outbursts, there were fights, shouts, and tussles during the whole waking day. Suicidal patients might be kept together and put in the care of a single nurse, charged with keeping them under constant and rigid surveillance and unable to allow any member of his sorry group any privacy. Patients in catatonic excitement would be confined to the padded room or a bare side-room until the phase passed. Hypomanic patients would pester and incite the others until trouble started, when they moved on to provoke someone else. The staff were hampered constantly by the knowledge that the bulk of their patients had failed to respond to all the treatments then available, and that therefore the outlook had to be accepted as hopeless, and the work as essentially custodial.

The advent of a drug that calmed without inducing sleep was obviously of great benefit in wards such as those described above. When, contrary to all expectations, the administration of the drug was sometimes found to coincide with a disappearance of positive schizophrenic symptoms and, less commonly but still more remarkably, the induction of warmth and spontaneity into previously withdrawn and unapproachable patients, the atmo-sphere in the chronic wards underwent a great and lasting change.

One of the most interesting and curious facets of the overall improvements in patients' behaviour and symptoms was that this improvement was not confined to those who had received the drug; the untreated patients benefited from the altered atmosphere, as even the most withdrawn patients always did in the distant past when chains were struck off or strait-jackets abolished. The newly activated patients, and those whose reduced symptoms allowed them to occupy themselves usefully, required and received rehabilitation and personal attention and guidance by nurses.

This attention led to further improvement, as did the more frequent attendances by doctors faced with the welcome neces-sity of assessing improvement and adjusting dosage. Patients who had been incontinent regained control of their functions, and destructive patients stopped trying to tear their clothes; the asylum suits became outmoded and patients were given or induced their relatives to bring them better clothes, regaining an interest in their appearance that many might have forgotten they ever possessed, and subsequently making further progress.

With many of the patients now looking normal and acting with superficial rationality for much of the time, the décor of the wards, many of them unchanged since the nineteenth century, was seen to be not only gloomy and depressing but incongruous; the use – tentative at first – of bright colours and furniture approximating in design and standard to that seen in modern homes served not only to take the patient one step further but encouraged disheartened relatives to resume the visiting they had neglected because it had been so depressing and, in the absence of any emotional response or expression of gratitude from the patient, purposeless. Each improvement in the régime seemed to react favourably on the patient, and it was the conservatism of hospital staffs and the shortage of funds rather than the gradual nature of the clinical response that dictated the speed at which the reforms were put under way; rumours even started to circulate that some mental hospitals were unlocking their doors.

The only disadvantage, or apparent disadvantage, of this chain-reaction was that it was no longer possible to say what were the precise effects of the new drugs. Because of the efforts of the drug industry to produce saleable drugs to which the name 'tranquillizer' could be appended, it became immediately important to distinguish pharmacologically induced remission from the secondary effects of improved environment and therapeutic optimism.

By the mid-fifties dozens of drugs and drug-combinations were on the market as tension-reducers, and their evaluation was an urgent matter. The most widely known of these was probably meprobamate (Equanil, Miltown), a minor tranquillizer of little utility that was dispensed in enormous quantities over this period, but today most of the others have deservedly fallen into disuse. However, one of the drugs, reserpine, is still used as a major tranquillizer. In the early days, in some mental hospitals, it was prescribed even more frequently than chlorpromazine.

Rauwolfia serpentina the source of reserpine, is a plant indigenous to India, where the powdered whole root has long had a reputation for efficacy in the treatment of a variety of ills, including psychiatric states. The crude preparation was used at first for its effect on raised blood-pressure, but in the late nineteen-forties the first occidental observation of its ability to render anxious patients 'tranquil' was recorded. In the early nineteen-fifties the marketing of the pure alkaloid, reserpine (Serpasil), enabled the drug to be given a psychiatric trial. Despite troublesome side-effects the agent seemed to have therapeutic possibilities corresponding approximately to those of chlorpromazine, and alone or in combination these drugs came to be the mainstay of anti-schizophrenic therapy.

The evaluation of these and other drugs took place under conditions so variable that even the preliminary planning of the drug trial (with the associated increase in interest among the nursing staff and the necessary examination of the patients' original mental states) resulted in overall improvement long before any actual medication was prescribed. One inevitable result was a closer examination of the therapeutic factors to which the patient responded and the methods that it was necessary to use in order that the results of the trial could be relied upon. It was quickly seen, most of all by the competing drug houses, that any drug given to long-neglected patients was liable to be reported as effective, and soon attention was focused on the drugs' *placebo effect* and the so-called *placebo-responders* of which a logical account is best given by referring once again to the past.

THE PLACEBO-RESPONDERS

Any therapy performed by a doctor is liable to make the patient believe that he is receiving purposeful treatment, and is usually attended by improvement. In the special case where the treatment is scientifically useless this beneficial effect, which follows with gratifying frequency, is called a placebo-effect and the treatment a placebo. All surgeons know that a purely exploratory abdominal operation, disclosing no disease, may well lead to a reduction in the symptoms of which the patient complained, while many, perhaps all, who practise psychotherapy, must have had patients who improved suddenly and lastingly while the therapist was still trying to get his bearings in the maze. Such of these improvements as cannot be accounted for by spontaneous cure must be due to the patient's response to a placebo. Both psychotherapy and surgery are or should be deemed too cumbersome and hazardous for routine use as placebos, however, and the most common type of placebos are pills and medicines. Even genuinely effective medicine exerts a placebo effect on top of its pharmacological action; many patients who cannot do without a sleeping pill drop off so quickly after taking their sedative that the onset of sleep precedes any possible significant response to the drug.

Until late in the history of medicine almost all drugs were placebos, and thus almost all therapeutic benefit occurred despite the objective inefficacy (and occasionally the toxic properties) of the drugs. Patients as well as doctors were dimly aware of this fact: the patients joked about the colour of the medicine the doctor gave them that week, and relished its bitterness while appreciating the purpose of the flavour; the doctors quoted the old saw about using new remedies quickly while they still continued to work, and applied the principle implicit in the saying by thinking as little as possible about the placebo-effect of drugs in order that they might believe in their own treatments and, by contagion, help their patients.

In the seventeenth century quinine, the first really effective remedy, was discovered and used for a variety of fevers for one of which, malaria, it was specific. Slowly and gradually other specific drugs followed, but until the sulphonamides and such antibiotics as penicillin gave physicians the necessary self-confidence they were slow to examine the placebo factors in their treatments (though occasionally willing to point them out in treatments used by other doctors or by lay groups like the osteopaths) on the sensible grounds that to do so would be tantamount to tearing up the *Pharmacopoeia*.

Even before the great advances of the nineteen-forties one group of doctors, the anaesthetists, were in the happy position of possessing enough effective drugs for their immediate purposes, and could examine the placebo-effect without detriment to their therapeutic powers; some exploited their observations that under the right circumstances the anxious patient could be rendered anaesthetic without the administration of significant quantities of drug by enhancing the impact of the surroundings and the doctor's presence in a way that amounted to the use of hypnotism. Others, notably at Harvard under Professor H. K. Beecher, studied the placebo quantitatively, with special reference to its effectiveness against pain. In general, it was found that more than a third of patients suffering pain responded satisfactorily to inactive drugs; and that a variety of symptoms responded in about the same proportion of patients, with the proviso that if the group were anxious more patients responded, while if the level of anxiety was low, for example in a strictly experimental situation where the participants knew that the induced pain they were experiencing was ultimately going to be terminated by the experimenter, less patients made a placebo-response. It was also found over a series of experiments that, as Arthur Shapiro pointed out in a widely quoted account of placebos, the ideal pill was as red as possible, as bitter as was compatible with ingesting it successfully, as complicated to take as possible (i.e. take two pills with one third of a glass of lukewarm water six minutes before each main meal, except on Tuesdays) and as unlike the familiar aspirin tablet as the maker could manage.

Psychiatrists were late to take serious interest in the placebo-effects and in the patients who consistently showed benefits from inert drugs, the placebo-responders, partly because the speciality was late in obtaining a respectable body of effective treatments but also, by way of corollary, because psychiatrists exploited placebo-effects most blatantly of all. These factors apart, psychiatrists were in a good position to examine the phenomenon: they were acutely aware of and in process of attempting to analyse the relationship between doctor and patient, a relationship they realized must have been all-important in producing temporary success for long-abandoned but once lauded treatments like mesmerism, auto-suggestion, and purging. The advent of tranquillizing drugs, which may be said to have promoted psychiatrists to physicians in the eyes of some of their colleagues, and the insane to the status of patients in the eyes of many members of the public, precipitated a considerable research effort into placebo-effects and many other aspects of the trial of new and allegedly useful remedies.

Physicians who are trying out drugs seldom or never do so entirely at random; they believe, on scientific or emotional grounds, that the drug has at least a fair chance of working, and whether the grounds themselves may be rationally formulated or not, the belief held by the physician concerned alters his subjective judgement; scientific training probably does not significantly modify this alteration, though it makes the physician more ready to admit to and allow for it. Therefore the method that is customarily used is one of assessing the patient's progress, as far as possible, by objective means such as the course of the temperature, the pulse, or the blood-pressure.

Even with illnesses of such seemingly clear-cut causation, course, and treatment as pneumonia these precautions, though they may be all that can be taken, are not entirely adequate; the doctor, by his optimism, may affect the patient's course as a good nurse would in the days when the management of pneumonia from its presentation to its crisis was almost entirely a nursing problem; and he may, by unusually frequent attentions and ministrations, cause the patient's chances to improve in a way analogous to that seen in animal experiments where rats that have been frequently handled display greater resistance to illness than those whose contact with their keepers has been less intimate.

In psychiatric work objectivity, though desirable and no doubt ultimately attainable, is seldom feasible in experiments done on the effectiveness of drugs. An objective rating-scale, corresponding to, say, a temperature chart in general medical work, might record the patient's day-to-day activity, food intake, social adaptability, conformity to the simple ward rules, and so on. Such rating scales, though widely used in trials because of their approach to objectivity, are too coarse to

measure many of the improvements noted as definite and striking when the patients are interviewed. Reliance on interview
assessments of patients' current mental states brings the problem of the placebo-responder into sharp focus. In psychiatric
practice the doctor–patient relationship, on which the placebo-
effect must depend, is assiduously cultivated; and though the
psychiatric patients most freely subjected to drug trials – the
chronic schizophrenics – are largely free from overt anxiety
about their states, and so far removed from normal patterns of
attitudes as sometimes to react better to a sweet rather than a
bitter medicine, the results of any interviews which purport to
measure the degree of improvement, if any, after the administration of a favoured drug must be strongly affected by the
psychiatrist's expectations and the reflection of these in his
patients' responses.

Investigations have shown that the patient who responds to
one placebo is likely to respond to another. The placebo-
responder, as a person, is likely to be extraverted, cooperative,
and uncomplaining compared with his fellows while his illness is
likely to include unelaborated anxiety among its symptoms. His
personality and symptom-complex are not distinctive enough,
however, for him to be recognized in advance and excluded from
a trial of drugs.

These considerations were highly relevant in the mid
nineteen-fifties because of the sudden and acute need to make
scientific assessments of many different drugs, all labelled
tranquillizers, all mysterious in their operation, and all producing a certain amount of apparent benefit in the groups of
patients to whom they were given. It was important that the
effective agents should be singled out so that the limited
resources available for research at the level of skill required
should be focused on the active drugs. To get round the
difficulties inherent in testing out remedies on patients whose
response, placebo or otherwise, was measured by the subjective
judgements of deeply interested doctors, a new methodology
was devised, derived in part from long-established experimental
principles but reaching, in psychiatric work, a greater pitch of
refinement: the methodology of drug trials. Because of the

great interest psychiatrists now have in the methods used, and the important results of the cooperation of clinicians and research pharmacologists in scientifically planned trials, a short account will be given of the general approach used before further developments in psychopharmacology are detailed.

DRUG TRIALS

A large manufacturer of medical drugs with a flourishing department of psychopharmacology may synthesize a dozen new compounds a month. Of these a proportion will show promise when coarse screening tests with animal subjects are applied. At the end of further screening tests, mostly designed to see if the drugs' actions correspond fairly closely to those of known tranquillizers, particularly those of chlorpromazine, three or four a year may be encouraging enough to seem to warrant further trial on humans. The stage at which it becomes necessary to use human subjects, if psychopharmacology is the field, is an early one, for no animals undergo any recognizable form of the major human psychoses of depression and schizophrenia, and the estimation of such subtle changes as a swing from mild depression to mild elation in a rat must be so subjective and intuitive (though it is attempted) as to make interview-assessment of a human patient a triumph of objectivity by comparison.

If there is evidence that a drug possesses new properties or signal advantages over known treatments for the condition for which it is envisaged, if there is no completely satisfactory remedy already available for the condition, and if toxicity trials in animals, during which disproportionately large quantities of the drug have been used for long periods of time, are reassuring, the manufacturer tries to arrange a clinical trial. Understandably, having invested considerable sums of money and many months of work, he is anxious that he should have some preliminary report as quickly as possible. His difficulty lies in finding doctors who are willing to undertake the work, and the reasons for medical reluctance at this stage are easy to understand.

The preliminary drug-trial involves a search for several factors, including the therapeutic effects, the side-effects, the toxic effects, and the ideal dosage and course of treatment. Work of this kind is exacting, expensive, and time-consuming, and cannot, if done conscientiously, be fitted into the routine of a busy hospital psychiatrist if neither his work nor the quality of his observations is to suffer: university and teaching centres, where the work could be more easily undertaken, are too few to handle trials of all the new remedies proffered. Furthermore, the chances of anything exciting or truly novel emerging from the results are small. Most of the host of new drugs produced in one year are forgotten by the next, while the chances of stumbling on serious toxicity are not negligible. Several psychopharmacological drugs have caused fatal and otherwise disastrous effects before being precipitately withdrawn from the market.

At the present time the situation is serious enough for the clinicians and pharmacologists to be considering setting up a 'clearing-house' for drug-trials: drugs will be screened for the qualities mentioned earlier, and the best will be offered, with the seal of approval of the screening-committee, to such hospitals and units as have expressed interest in conducting drug-trials at this stage. This arrangement will, it is hoped, relieve doctors of pressure from the drug firms to try out their new products while at the same time ensuring that what seem to be the best of these are carefully and thoroughly examined, once and for all. Advances in animal experiment will lessen the need for elaborate preliminary or pilot trials, with their inevitable risks. It goes without saying that such trials are done only on patients refractory to other remedies or in some way intolerant of them, and that the patients are fully informed of the nature of the procedures and their implications during the experiment.

Drugs that survive the pilot trial are then subjected to a somewhat complex formal assessment. The details and the particular experimental designs used vary with investigators and diseases but the overall pattern is constant. Let us suppose that a new tranquillizer is to be tested. Data available include the usual dosage, the probable side-effects, the disease entity on which it is hoped it may act, and the benefits noted in the pilot trial as likely to result.

First, patients with the disease in question are selected. Ideally the selection is done by psychiatrists not concerned in the trial itself, and the patients are diagnosed separately by each psychiatrist, only those for whom diagnoses coincide being included: this ensures that the group is homogeneous for the illness and that possible therapeutic benefit in schizophrenia is not obscured by contamination with the drug's effects on, say, depression, which may be different and undesirable.

Next the patients are randomly divided into two groups. The members of the first group will receive the active drug and members of the second the inert drug or placebo, made up in such a manner that its appearance is identical; the purpose of this division is to arrange that the placebo-effect which will undoubtedly occur will be manifest in both groups of patients, so that any statistically significant difference between the overall progress of one group and that of the other will be fairly attributable to the strictly pharmacological activity of the drug. Because statistical significance may be achieved with smaller numbers or with less finely differing results if the technique is somewhat modified by 'pairing', the trial is sometimes designed in such a way that each patient in the first group has a partner, similar in certain respects to himself, in the second. Experimental trials of this kind are called 'controlled', the group receiving the active drug being known as the experimental group and those receiving the placebo as the control group.

Where the drug's effects are likely to continue only for as long as the drug continues to act within the body, and where the disease is one that persists in the absence of treatment – as would be the case with the trial of a new tranquillizer in a group of chronic schizophrenics – each patient in the trial may be made to act as his own control if the members of the experimental group receive the active drug for a period of, say, six weeks, following which they receive placebo; with the control group of the first six weeks following a reverse course. The plan described is that of a 'blind' trial, in which the patients are unaware of the contents of the tablets they receive. If each patient acts as his own control by receiving active drug at one stage of the experiment and placebo at another, it becomes a blind 'crossover' trial.

The precautions taken so far would not be sufficient if the doctors assessing the patients' progress knew which subjects were currently receiving active tablets; it must be assumed, and is generally agreed, that their therapeutic enthusiasm would influence both the patients' responses and the interviewer's assessment of these. The drugs are therefore dispensed in accordance with a prearranged code by the hospital pharmacist, who alone knows which patient is getting active and which inert tablets. When this plan is followed the experiment is called a 'double blind' controlled crossover trial, and this is the commonest form of informative trial done in hospitals today.

It may be modified to compare a new drug with a standard drug such as chlorpromazine, or to compare three or four different drugs, or to cover several hospitals and their staffs where the condition involved is rare and no hospital can provide adequate subjects on its own, or where very large numbers are needed because of the subtlety of the differences expected.

In the planning of the more complicated trials and in the analysis of the results statistical advice may be invaluable: the use of statistical methods enables the results to be judged as probably significant and meaningful, or as probably due to chance. Ideally the calculations are done before the code is broken.

This elaborate kind of trial has the disadvantages of being cumbersome, exacting, and rigid. If patients react differently from the manner expected their reactions may not fit into the categories to which attention is being paid. If any patient falls ill it may become necessary to break the code and find out if he is receiving the active drug. Both these faults emphasize the need for thorough preliminary trial. The advantages of this type of controlled trial in weeding out drugs that had no true usefulness were epitomized by G. A. Foulds, who pointed out in a lively article that of seventy-two British and American trials, both adequately controlled and uncontrolled, reported in and randomly selected from psychiatric journals, only 25 per cent of

the controlled trials showed the drug helpful, while the uncontrolled work purported to show success in more than 75
per cent. Certainly, since these trials have been used widely,
most of the early tranquillizers have fallen by the wayside, and
the actions of the effective agents have been more accurately
described. Reference will be made to trials of this kind later in
this chapter and throughout the book, and their impact on the
status of long-established treatments such as deep insulin
(coma) treatment is discussed in the appropriate chapters.

Finally, the trial of the drug is completed by its steady use in
medicine; here the general practitioner is the most helpful
observer. Drugs may be free from acute deleterious side-effects,
and they may be potent therapeutically, and yet still display
serious toxicity after prolonged use or in unusual circumstances:
because of their chronic (long-term) ill-effects, pheniprazine
(Cavodil) and etryptamine (Monase) have been withdrawn from
the market after years of use; the effects of certain other drugs on
the developing foetus have led to their withdrawal, or to
restrictions on their use during pregnancy.

FURTHER DEVELOPMENTS IN CHEMOTHERAPY

As reliable knowledge of the range of usefulness of tranquillizers accumulated, and as the chemical field was narrowed
down to the phenothiazine molecule and its congeners, considerable advances, albeit gradual, were made. Drugs such as
trifluoperazine (Stelazine) and prochlorperazine (Stemetil),
possessing anti-psychotic potency equalling though probably
not surpassing that of chlorpromazine (which remains for
most psychiatrists their drug of choice) and differing helpfully
in their detailed effects, were marketed. Interesting agents,
often of theoretical rather than clinical value, based on the
phenothiazine molecule were found, with effects as diverse as
couch-suppression, diuresis, and the relief of pain.

Toxicity, sometimes of a peculiarly disquieting kind such as
retinal damage, was also reported in a number of drugs at preliminary stages of investigation. The thorough and reliable

testing of the drugs enabled the chemists and pharmacologists to work out suitable animal screening tests, and attempts were made to relate the differing actions of the various phenothiazine drugs tested to the dissimilarities in their structure. This task of determining structure-activity relationship (S.A.R.) has made some progress of an empirical kind, but since the way in which the phenothiazines act is unknown, no comprehensive explanation of the variation of pharmacology with structure is impending at present.

The chemists and pharmacologists, in an attempt to better the activity of chlorpromazine, have synthesized and tested a large number of drugs. To some extent the prospects of anything radically new being found were lessened by the organization of the investigations done on the drugs produced, since this had been fashioned around chlorpromazine. It followed that any novel actions of a tranquillizer would probably be found in clinical pilot trials, and then only by a doctor who was not blinkered by past experience. The next discovery, made in just this way, was to start another spurt in the serious game of molecular manipulation.

THE ANTI-DEPRESSIVE DRUGS

In 1950 the Swiss drug firm Geigy invited R. Kuhn to investigate a compound later called imipramine, which was a product of a line of research differing from the usual one of substituting new side-chains on the phenothiazine molecule. In this instance, the sulphur atom was removed from the phenothiazine nucleus and replaced by a two-carbon bridge; the compound, in its action on animals, resembled chlorpromazine fairly closely, and its clinical trial took the form of testing it for corresponding therapeutic results. Kuhn presumably found little of interest in its action, for he abandoned work on it for a period of four years, after which he undertook further trials of this and other iminodibenzyl derivatives.

Over the ensuing three years about five hundred patients were treated with these 'tranquillizers', but the most important fact that came out in Kuhn's paper was not concerned with schizophrenic symptomatology. He noted instead that imipramine specifically and sometimes rather dramatically relieved psychotic depression. It was thus the first drug to reflect in its action the anti-depressive effect of electro-convulsive therapy (see Chapter 3). Geigy marketed this drug as Tofranil, and it has been extensively employed in the treatment of depressive illnesses, particularly those of the so-called endogenous group.

Until Tofranil became available only electro-convulsive therapy could be offered to shorten the depressive illness, which meant that illnesses too severe to respond to symptomatic medication of a sedative kind and either not severe enough to warrant electro-convulsive therapy or untreated because the patient refused to undergo the treatment, could not be helped. At present, the drug may be used alone in the treatment of illnesses that previously could not conveniently receive electro-convulsive therapy, while it may also be used as an adjunct to electrical treatment to reduce the chance of post-treatment relapse. The most interesting aspect of Tofranil's effect on depression, which becomes apparent only after a lag of a week or two and is only seen in about 60 per cent of patients treated, was the promise inherent in the drug: it seemed and seems inevitable that a drug will be found that works both more promptly and more regularly.

In order that they should bring this happy discovery about, the drug firms re-examined the pharmacology of imipramine (Tofranil), and made further studies of the structure-activity relationships involved. Unfortunately for these researches the most definite difference between imipramine and chlorpromazine seemed to be the anti-depressive effect itself; used in animals, the drug acted like a tranquillizer, i.e. like a potentially anti-schizophrenic agent. As indicated previously, this was probably in part the result of relying on tests developed when testing the chlorpromazine family, but it is not easy to see what other tests could be applied: the rat does not suffer from melancholia, so far as is known, and minor improvements in its mood cannot be discerned.

In this dilemma the pharmacologists exploited knowledge gained by clinicians in a different setting. It will be remembered that the Indian remedy from which reserpine was derived had undergone trial, with some success, in the treatment of schizophrenia. It had also been used to counteract hypertension (high blood-pressure). A small proportion of the patients who took this drug over a long period of time developed a classical depressive illness, and it was recognized that depression, sometimes of suicidal severity, was an occasional long-term toxic effect of reserpine. The pharmacologists experimentally determined one action of Tofranil that might be linked with its anti-depressive activity by showing that it would counteract the effects of reserpine on the rabbit in a manner which chlorpromazine, so like it in other pharmacological ways, would not. In the screening of new compounds reserpine-antagonism is now becoming a routine procedure, but there is no guarantee, and indeed it is unlikely, that reserpine-antagonism in the case of a rabbit really corresponds with the treatment in the human of the depressive illness occasionally associated with chronic reserpine medication. The unsatisfactory state of pharmacological tests done on animals will be referred to again when theoretical considerations are reviewed.

Consideration of the structure-activity relationships, superficial though it necessarily was, indicated that if chlorpromazine could be changed into an anti-depressive compound by the substitution of a two-carbon bridge for the sulphur in the phenothiazine ring, then an analogue of chlorpromazine with more sedative effect might, if manipulated in a similar manner, produce an anti-depressive drug also – perhaps with rather more sedative effect. This ingenious parallel led to the production of a second useful compound, amitriptyline (Tryptizol), which is now also in general use for the treatment of depressions, particularly those associated with agitation and anxiety.

So far in this account, several drugs (chlorpromazine and its cousins, and imipramine and amitriptyline) have been described, which are unique in psychiatric treatment and which have between them changed the whole pattern of treatment of psychoses, both in hospital and at home. Yet there is something seemingly unscientific about the manner in which the discoveries were made. Chlorpromazine was recognized as an anti-psychotic agent when the pharmacologists were looking for something else; imipramine was noted to be an anti-depressive in the course of an anti-schizophrenic trial. Nobody was more aware of the inadequacy of the theoretical background than the chemists and the psychiatrists who were wondering where to go next, especially since, far from entering into predictions, they could not even explain the observed facts. Help was to come from an unexpected quarter, though the manner in which it came (a chance observation of a side-effect of a drug being used for a totally different purpose) was all too familiar.

THE MONOAMINE OXIDASE INHIBITORS

In 1955 tuberculosis was starting to respond to the isolation of infective patients in sanatoria; the corresponding reduction in the pool of infective patients in the community was leading to a fall in the incidence of the disease. At the same time the patients already infected were being treated with three main anti-tubercular drugs as well as undergoing their long régime of rest and fresh air. These drugs, an antibiotic called strepto-mycin, and two synthetic agents called para-aminosalicylic acid (P.A.S.) and isoniazid, were not ideal because they were not toxic enough to the bacterium and were sometimes too toxic to the patient; but their main drawback was that the tubercle bacilli were liable to develop resistance to the drugs.

Isoniazid, one of the most effective of the anti-tubercular drugs, was itself the product of molecular manipulation and, in common with the other agents, soon produced strains of tubercle bacilli which were resistant to its effects. Among its advantages was its ease of administration: streptomycin had to be given by injection, while P.A.S. was bulky and unpleasant to take. Isoniazid was both active and pleasant, and when it was first tried out it produced in the patients who received it a marked and sometimes troublesome elevation of mood.

Interestingly enough, investigation of this response showed that it was simply the expression of the comprehensible joy of patients whose hopes had been justifiably raised; the negative results of this investigation fortunately did not inhibit later investigators after the next step was taken. Because of the frequent occurrence of isoniazid-resistant tubercle bacilli, a similar substance, the isopropyl congener called *iproniazid*, was given a clinical trial. Once again euphoria resulted, but on this occasion investigation of the psychic effects showed that they could not be accounted for in terms of comprehensible and appropriate joy: a potent anti-depressive drug had been found. Not only that, but a clue was provided as to the possible means of action, for pharmacological studies had already shown that iproniazid, unlike the earlier isoniazid, was an inhibitor of a certain enzyme, known to be of importance in the metabolism of such hormones as adrenaline, called monoamine oxidase.

The drug, given the trade-name of Marsilid, was tried out on psychiatric patients in 1956 and many articles soon testified to its promising effects. Controlled trials, while tempering this enthusiasm, were sufficiently encouraging to make study of other monoamine oxidase inhibitors worth while, and soon three other drugs were on the market – nialamide (Niamid), phenelzine (Nardil), and pheniprazine (Cavodil).

All these drugs produced an improvement in the mood of a proportion of the patients to whom they were given. Their long-term toxicity, as experience proved, was formidable, and pheniprazine (Cavodil) has been withdrawn, while iproniazid (Marsilid) is regarded in many centres as too toxic for use. Further monoamine oxidase inhibitors (isocarboxazid or Marplan; tranylcypromine or Parnate) have taken their place, but liver-damage seems rather consistently to be associated with the hydrazine molecule and the capacity to inhibit monoamine oxidase, and this group of drugs does not in general provide a therapeutic method as safe as that of Tofranil or electrical treatment.

Nevertheless, as previously indicated, these agents did seem to give a lead to the proximate chemistry of mood. An enzyme like monoamine oxidase is an organic catalyst, a substance that speeds a chemical reaction without itself taking part in the main chemical changes. Without such enzymes chemical reactions in the cells of the body would, like chemical reactions in

industrial plants in the absence of catalysts, become un-
economically slowed. It was reasoned that if some such drug as
iproniazid inhibited monoamine oxidase, then whatever substance it was that monoamine oxidase broke down would
increase in quantity; and that an increase in the quantity of the
substance, if associated with an elevation of mood, argued that
the substance might itself be the arbiter of mood: a veritable
humour at last.

The question was, what was the substance? One answer was
quickly provided. For years, a substance called *serotonin* had
been under intense scrutiny by pharmacologists and biochemists. It was first described as a factor in serum which maintained the tone in the walls of small blood vessels (hence the
name) and analysis showed that it was a relatively simple compound, 5-hydroxytryptamine. Numerous subsequent publica-
tions told of its wide distribution – in platelets, certain tumours,
the central nervous system, and banana pulp. By 1957 Uden-
friend and his collaborators could write, 'That serotonin is an
important agent can no longer be questioned. It remains now
to determine exactly where and how it functions.' (It is comforting to find that it is not psychiatrists alone who follow this
order.) The most significant facts for those interested in the
central nervous system were that reserpine (the drug that sometimes induces depression) displaced serotonin from its natural
sites, including those in the brain, or prevented it being taken
up, that serotonin was probably concerned in mediation at the
junction of nerves; and that in its free form it was susceptible to
the action of the enzyme monoamine oxidase. It was therefore
an immediate and obvious candidate for the role of the chemical
mediator of mood, and research on the substance was given fresh
impetus.

By virtue of its simplicity and unitary nature the *serotonin
hypothesis* was popular with psychiatrists (whose optimism
seems inexhaustible), but it soon proved too simple to be maintained. It is now recognized that the serotonin levels in the brain
are not so closely associated with mood change as those of the
less novel agents, adrenaline and nor-adrenaline (the catechol-
amines), which are also degraded by monoamine oxidase.

What is clear, however, is that the biochemists, pharmacologists, and experimentally inclined psychiatrists are circling in the right area. Serotonin has intimate connexions with the actions of reserpine; it is also an antagonist to L.S.D., a drug which produces an artificial psychosis in man. Adrenaline and nor-adrenaline are agents associated with the fear responses of human beings and seem also, as just described, to have a close relationship to mood. Tofranil, the anti-depressive agent developed from the tranquillizers, is a reserpine antagonist, and may sensitize nerve-junctions in the brain to the actions of adrenaline, thus producing a corresponding functional effect to that of the monoamine oxidase inhibitors. All these findings must in some way be connected, but our knowledge of the anatomical and functional organization of the brain is as yet too poor to show how. Because of the inaccessibility of the parts under study, advance in this basic understanding can only be slow.

THE STATUS OF DRUGS IN PSYCHIATRY TODAY

While the dramatic advances described above were taking place, progress was also being made in other directions. Many of the drugs (L.S.D., Antabuse, sex hormones, etc.) resulting from or popularized by such work as I have just described are limited and specialized in their application, and they will be described in the sections of this book devoted to the conditions for which they are most commonly used.

At the present time the standard method of treatment used in *acute schizophrenia* is the administration of chlorpromazine (Largactil) or some more recent tranquillizer in full dosage. Symptomatic treatment with sedatives and adjuvant treatment with electro-convulsive therapy may be used, but the hopes of eliminating the schizophrenic process rest on the phenothiazine drug. There is some difference of opinion about the true effect of the major tranquillizers. Some workers believe that their action is suppressive only, and that they are merely symptom-removing. Others, including myself, think on grounds of equal subjectivity that the best responses to phenothiazines so closely resemble complete cures as to be indistinguishable from them, and posit an action of the drug that is associated with reversal of the pathological process of schizophrenia.

Over the years the various phenothiazine drugs have been thoroughly tested: none of the major tranquillizers such as chlor-promazine, prochlorperazine, trifluoperazine, perphenazine, and thioridazine has any compelling advantage over its fellows, though the effectiveness of trifluoperazine in schizophrenic states with many hallucinations is sometimes extolled, and a certain drug may be more preferable with certain types of dominant symptoms because of its individual spectrum of activity. In general, psychiatrists sensibly use the drug to which they are most accustomed, turning to other drugs or to combinations of drugs if the first is not fully effective. The outlook in schizophrenia is variable, and the recent improvement in the outlook cannot be ascribed entirely to the use of phenothiazine drugs; in general terms, however (quoting figures provided by P. Rhode and W. Sargant), an acutely schizophrenic patient, treated reasonably early with full dosage of chlorpromazine, now stands a better than 70 per cent chance of great improvement or recovery within two months.

The *chronic schizophrenic*, ill for longer than two years, does less well: when phenothiazines were first used, a proportion of the chronic population of the mental hospitals made startling recoveries, but at the present time the phenothiazines and other major tranquillizers are only one item in the list of expedients used to encourage improvement in this group, and most psychiatrists would reckon them less important than social and administrative measures.

In the immediate management of the *disturbed and destructive* patient, of whatever diagnostic category, the phenothiazines used solely for the purpose of inducing tranquillity are valuable agents: it will be remembered that the employment of chlorpro-mazine for this purpose first drew attention to the value of the drug in psychiatry. In the agitated and confused states that may result from senile changes in the brain, and in the deliria associated with more acute disturbances of cerebral function secondary to fevers and intoxications, the phenothiazines are useful and may, by shortening or suppressing an exhausting mental state, be life-saving.

The phenothiazine molecule is not a simple one, and the phenothiazine drugs are potent agents. Consequently the use of the drugs is sometimes attended by allergic or hypersensitive reactions, and is invariably accompanied by side-effects. The individual toxic effects such as jaundice, blood disorders, and skin rashes usually necessitate the substitution of another drug; all these reactions, though serious and on rare occasions fatal, have been reported with the first of the phenothiazine tranquillizers, chlorpromazine; the drug is used in such enormous quantities, however, and serious toxicity is so uncommonly reported, that chlorpromazine and the other major tranquillizers may be regarded as relatively safe drugs.

The side-effects of the major tranquillizers follow a similar pattern: most of them may lead to excessive sedation, most have effects on the autonomic or vegetative nervous system, and most produce effects on the deep nuclei of the brain, leading usually to a reversible condition known as parkinsonism. These constant side-effects may be connected with the drug's mode of action, and the parkinsonism in particular has been the source of much speculation and interest.

In the treatment of *depressive states* drugs do not yet play the leading role. The depressed patient may need urgent treatment either for life-saving purposes if he is suicidal, or on humane grounds if his distress is, as it may be, well nigh intolerable. Though the drugs may be started at once because of the help they may provide after a week or two, they are not prompt enough in their action to be used alone, and are less frequently fully effective when used in depression of suicidal severity: most psychiatrists would prefer to employ electrical treatment in these circumstances, and indeed, in my opinion, might justifiably be criticized if they did not advise it.

For the patient with mild depression, or the patient who tends to relapse after electrical treatment, however, the anti-depressive drugs have proved a boon. Imipramine (Tofranil) in particular may produce improvement of a very convincing kind after a week or so, and all the anti-depressive drugs mentioned in this chapter elevate mood significantly in about 50 per cent of the patients who receive them. For the endogenous type of depression imipramine (Tofranil) is the drug of choice, with amitriptyline (Tryptizol) offering some special advantages if the patient is unusually agitated. For depressive states in general any of the monoamine oxidase inhibitors may be used, the choice of drug depending usually on the individual psychiatrist's experience and the information on the agent's toxicity currently available. Isocarboxazid (Marplan) seems relatively safe, and tranylcypromine (Parnate) though more hazardous, has also been widely used and seems to have a rapid therapeutic effect. With the anti-depressive drugs, as with the tranquillizers, the psychiatrist may ring the changes if he does not produce benefit with his first remedy; caution has to be exercised if imipramine is given immediately after a course of a monoamine oxidase inhibitor, because the effects of the latter drugs may linger on for two or three weeks and because, presumably as a consequence of related but incompatible modes of action, bizarre movements and collapse may, rarely, follow. Imipramine may be followed by amine oxidase inhibitors with less chance of similar disasters, probably because it is more promptly degraded in the body, and it is thus a frequent choice as the initial drug.

The toxic and side-effects of the anti-depressive drugs have been more alarming than those of the tranquillizers. Imipramine is relatively safe, its most notable toxic action being an extension of its therapeutic action, when it causes a patient to over-swing from depression to a state of pathological elation; experience in the use of the drug has reduced the incidence of hypomanic episodes of this kind. Its side-effects are tiresome and uncomfortable, including a dry mouth, tremor, flushing, impotence, and constipation, but are usually tolerated by a depressed patient if he knows that a reasonable prospect of improvement exists. The monoamine oxidase inhibitors, most of which stem from the hydrazine molecule, lead sometimes to liver damage of a severe and not infrequently fatal variety: their side-effects are variable, but not usually severe; they too may lead to hypomanic reactions and because of the slow onset and wearing off of the drugs' effects these reactions may be hard to foresee and to control.

In the treatment of *psychoneurotic states* the main emphasis is on psychotherapy and, where possible, alteration of the environment in an attempt to modify the stresses operating on the patient; but some psychoneuroses such as obsessive-compulsive neurosis may resist these measures, while others may respond more readily if the overall level of anxiety is reduced. The major tranquillizers have no place in the treatment of psychoneurotic anxiety; not only may the drugs be expected to cause toxic effects in a small proportion of patients, effects that must be weighed against the comparatively minor nature of psychoneurotic illnesses, but unwelcome psychological effects may ensue. Minor tranquillizers, such as the phenothiazine promazine, or the well-known meprobamate (Equanil) are of some use, and a more recent drug called chlordiazepoxide (Librium) has been adequately proved, but it is doubtful whether, on balance, they have distinct advantages over the well-tried and virtually non-toxic amylobarbitone (Amytal).

Both tranquillizers and monoamine oxidase inhibitors have been used in the treatment of *severe or chronic pain*. In part, they work by potentiating the effect of the pain-killing drugs, but they may also have an independent effect on the patient's attitude to the pain or his capacity to register it. In the treatment of pain the placebo effect is often at its most prominent. Controlled series have not borne out some of the earlier claims but the agents are worth trying in certain conditions – those, for instance, that are so painful that even leucotomy may be invoked.

THE PROSPECTS FOR CHEMOTHERAPY

The account, given earlier in this chapter, of the manner in which the important discoveries of the last decade were made must not be allowed to disguise the high quality of the work that has been done. The alliance of chemist, pharmacologist, and clinical observer has proved formidable and productive.

It is to be expected that theoretical advances will offer some guidance to chemists in future years (though, as I have mentioned in another context (see p. 90), it would be too optimistic to expect that within a short while the chemical, electrical, and psychological organization of the brain will be completely discovered). Even without such assistance the process of molecular manipulation will continue to produce new drugs. The screening of new substances by means of animal tests is at present rather primitive in spite of the elegance of the experiments themselves, but this defect, with its wasteful consequences, is under urgent examination by the commercial drug-firms. With better screening and more rationally organized pilot trials on human patients, such therapeutic opportunities as the laboratories' efforts offer should be more readily seized.

The tendency, slow but sure, towards early exploitation of the informative methods of controlled double-blind trials does not only mean that the effective agents will be selected from the ineffective at an early date. It also means that useless remedies will not be used for long periods, distracting attention from truly useful drugs and multiplying the possibilities of long-term toxicity, simply *in case* they are effective and in case withholding them would deprive the patient of possible benefit.

There seems no reason why the manifestations of delirium, of pathological elation, of depression, and of morbid anxiety, already susceptible to amelioration, should not ultimately yield consistently to new and improved drugs, since drugs are already known that may induce these states. Whether depression will ever respond to drugs in the same way that it does to electrical treatment is less apparent. Schizophrenia, the illness of which the prognosis seemed most radically altered by the new drugs, is still far from mastered. Yet, to adopt an attitude of faith in the face of such a vast field of unknowns, even this illness must surely soon be overcome.

The Current Role of
Physical Treatment

3

Physical treatments, as the name implies, are those in which psychological symptoms are influenced by some means other than the spiritual, intellectual, and emotional pressures brought to bear in psychotherapy or the replacement of an unsuitable environment by one more calculated to encourage the patient to activity of a helpful kind. Though the term strictly includes chemotherapeutic treatment with drugs such as Largactil, it is conventionally applied only to treatments like insulin coma therapy and electric treatment, the so-called 'shock' therapies. The term 'shock treatment' is allowable because insulin coma therapy was rationalized, though not instituted, as a means of giving imperfectly operating neurons a cellular shock or metabolic jolt, while electric treatment (electro-convulsive therapy, E.C.T., electroplexy) is, of course, administered by means of an electric shock. But it is regrettable that the treatments have come to be equated, in the minds not only of potential patients but of some doctors, with such cruel psychological 'shock' treatments as the ancients used when they attempted to frighten the senses back into the deranged. To the unsophisticated but sane person the archaic shock methods may have a certain attraction and paradoxical sense, unless he falls ill and needs treatment himself. If he then includes electric treatment in the same quasi-punitive group in his own mind, as he well may because of the verbal coincidence, he is not likely to welcome the suggestion that he should receive it. It has been observed that psychiatrists may be happy to receive shock treatment when they are ill, but the public becomes Freudian to a man, distrusting the name, the idea, and its implications.

It is best to state at the outset that physical treatments are used because they work. They frequently come under fire from psychiatrists whose theoretical standpoint is that they ought not to, but those who use these treatments do not do so on theoretical grounds (because no satisfactory explanation of their effectiveness exists) but empirically. The treatments are best understood by considering their separate modes of development.

ELECTRIC TREATMENT

In 1935 von Meduna noted that schizophrenics did not commonly suffer from epilepsy, while epileptics had relative freedom from schizophrenia. On the basis of this observation, which later turned out to be incorrect, he decided to try the effects of a cerebral stimulant which was known to produce epileptic fits when given in toxic doses. He had accurately remarked the occasional improvement shown by the schizophrenic who was also epileptic, after a spontaneous fit. Accordingly, von Meduna injected cerebral stimulants intravenously, causing the patient greater and greater agitation as the level in the blood rose, until a fit caused loss of consciousness. The method produced results promising enough, in those days of therapeutic bankruptcy, to force psychiatrists to continue its use, but probably no treatment has ever engendered so much fear in the hearts of those receiving it. One frivolous theory about its effectiveness was that it was so terrifying that even the psychotic would deny his symptoms to get off the treatment list; but injections that produced fear without a fit brought about no benefit. In 1937–8 the method of producing fits by the brief passage of an electric current across the temples was introduced by Cerletti and Bini, and the treatment of psychosis by convulsions became at once less cumbersome and more humane.

At about the same time it was observed that of those given this anti-schizophrenic treatment the patients who did best were the ones who had been misdiagnosed, i.e. those who were not schizophrenic at all; and the treatment turned out to be specific for the other great functional psychosis, depression.

Since that time the treatment has been refined by the simultaneous use of anaesthetics and its indications have been more precisely determined, but the essence of the therapy – the administration of repeated fits – remains unchanged. Despite its specificity, negligible mortality, and wide use, the treatment has certain serious disadvantages: for example, it produces a transient memory difficulty which may upset a patient who is already concerned about himself and may feel that his memory is specially vulnerable; it is not infrequently followed by a severe headache which may last for several hours; and it occasionally produces in patients a pronounced fear of the treatment that is unexplained and is out of all proportion to the triviality of the procedure. With suicide from depressive states constituting one of the major causes of death, the side-effects would have to be rather severe before electric treatment could be abandoned without something to put in its place. Though recently the anti-depressive drugs have made physicians hopeful that one day chemotherapy will replace electric treatment, the present drugs are far too slow and uncertain in their effects to supplant electric treatment in cases of suicidal depression. For most of the period during which electric treatment has been available there have been no anti-depressive drugs, and so much work has been done to try to so modify the treatment that its disadvantages are minimized.

At first the investigators concentrated on the type of apparatus and current used to precipitate the epileptic fit; many complex apparatuses were designed and tested, for which various advantages were claimed; in general these 'machines' were intended to produce a fit with the use of as small a current as possible, though some were designed to prevent the fit actually occurring, in the hope that the passage of electricity might in itself produce equal benefit. One of the best known of these modifications involved the passage of current over a period of several minutes without the production of a fit, and was called electronarcosis. Like all the variations failing to produce fits it gave poor therapeutic results and it was ultimately abandoned because it was found sometimes to lead to intellectual damage and even death. L. B. Kalinowsky and P. H. Hoch, reviewing the work done, correctly conclude that for a machine to be useful it must regularly induce a convulsion while, other things being equal, the simpler the machine and the less likely it is to break down, the better.

During the Second World War the use of short-acting intravenous anaesthetics such as thiopentone (Pentothal) became popular, the idea of using such a drug being to ease the patient's treatment by preventing him from experiencing alarm as the electrodes were applied. Later, when curare, a muscle-relaxant derived from the crude preparation used as arrow-poison, stimulated interest in the possibilities of synthetic muscle-relaxants, and succinyl choline (Scoline), a short-acting relaxant, was produced, it became customary in hospitals with the necessary facilities to use thiopentone and subsequent succinyl choline to render the patient unconscious and 'damp down' the muscular accompaniments of the fit. The general trend since the war has been towards modifying electric treatment in this manner, and lately an intravenous anaesthetic even briefer in its action than thiopentone, called methohexital (Brevital) has been on trial. The use of anaesthetic and relaxant, though it reduces the unpleasant outward signs of the fit and enables complete amnesia for the event to be assured, introduces the element of risk inevitably associated with the administration of anaesthetic drugs, and though the small chance of fractures is reduced by this method it is possible to argue that the objective disadvantages outweight the advantages in the long run.

The indications for electric treatment became firmly established during and after the Second World War. Its prime use is in the treatment of severe depression, when characteristically the patient may show some improvement after two treatments and himself remark upon the return of some early well-being after three. It may also be used to relieve the acutely schizophrenic patient of his dramatic and troublesome symptoms, thus aiding the management of the illness and enabling the patient to take the drugs on which his progress is expected to rely. Where the acute schizophrenic has a mood-change among his symptoms, it may be eradicated with electric treatment in the same way as with purely depressed patients.

The chronic schizophrenic may benefit from occasional

electric treatment which, if given with discrimination, can assist in keeping him free from fresh delusional ideas or up-surges of hallucinations; also it may counteract the patient's tendency to withdraw from social contact. The manic or hypomanic patient, showing symptoms that are the reverse of those seen in depression, needs more intensive electrical treatment than his depressed counterpart, and is more likely to relapse and need to resume his course. Occasionally electric treatment may be used to precipitate a fit in an epileptic who shows uncomfortable or distressing symptoms during the few days before a convulsion, the artificially induced fit ending the ordeal; and some therapists resort to electric treatment in the treatment of delirium, if this is exhausting and intractable.

Obviously, then, electric treatment has wide uses and is widely used. Despite its doubtful reputation, it is often life-saving, and the manner in which it can cut short the misery of melancholia is striking and memorable. Used by doctors versed in its indications, its beneficial effects can be predicted with an accuracy that is seldom matched in medicine even when venerable drugs such as digitalis and morphine are used.

Nevertheless, the treatment is not well-liked. Its many uses have meant that it has also many potential abuses, and though it is wrong to think of electric treatment as being a short-cut, or as a therapy used instead of psychotherapy when doctors are scarce, there has been a tendency, in overcrowded and under-doctored institutions, to use it too frequently on incompletely assessed patients. The distaste, amounting in some cases to a fixed revulsion, that some treated patients feel towards the procedure has not lessened notably, even though the process of being treated has been modified to the point where nothing is done until the patient is completely anaesthetized; it follows that this occasional antipathy must arise from something inherent in the treatment or its brief aftermath – the awakening with a reduction or temporary loss of memory, the sense of unreality sometimes described during the post-treatment period, or some other psychological sequel to the fit. There also exists the real disadvantage that some doctors, particularly in the U.S.A., and many vocal members of the community such as writers, regard the treatment as intrinsically wrong and entirely dispensable, and do not hesitate persuasively to say so.

It is fortunate then, no matter what theoretical or practical point of view one holds, that the indications for electrical treatment are gradually lessening, though as yet, because of the increasing provision of psychiatric services, the numbers of treatments given have probably not reached their peak. Most of the troublesome symptoms of acute schizophrenia, delirium, and mania can now be controlled by tranquillizers. Epileptics whose pre-fit period is disturbed are few, and become fewer as advances in anti-epileptic drugs occur. Those who need can receive electric treatment to antedate the fit they were building up to, when the treatment may be regarded as anticipatory rather than a radical intervention. In the treatment of severe depression, electric treatment remains supreme.

In the future it is likely that the advent of new anti-depressive drugs will make electric treatment as dispensable as some of its critics would say it is already. When the mood-elevating drugs imipramine (Tofranil) and iproniazid came on the market in the late nineteen-fifties there was a tendency to use them in place of electric treatment; but the consequent delay in improvement, increase in suicides and attempted suicides, and the failure in many patients to end the depressive illness led to a reconsideration of the available drugs, and a return to electric treatment for most of the endogenously depressed patients admitted to hospital. For the moment, then, this type of therapy remains a useful, perhaps for the seriously ill the single most useful, treatment: its theoretical implications will be touched upon later in this chapter.

INSULIN COMA THERAPY

Insulin is one of the active hormones secreted by the pancreas, and it is concerned in the metabolism of the substance glucose, the consequence of administering insulin being the reduction of the level of circulating glucose in the blood. In the common disease diabetes, the blood-sugar is raised for most or all of the time due to a lessened ability to metabolize glucose, a defect that may be largely remedied by the injection of insulin derived from animals. The isolation and, soon afterwards, the commercial preparation and medical use of insulin was one of the great biochemical and therapeutic advances of the nineteen-twenties. In common with other new agents of specific usefulness (thyroid, procaine, vitamins, etc.) this hormone was tried out on many patients whose illnesses, though they had nothing in common with that for which the drug was indicated, shared the property of being difficult to treat. Psychiatric patients were given trials of the hormone, and it was found that some relief of symptoms could be achieved if small doses of insulin were administered, the blood sugar was allowed to fall, and then a meal was given to raise the blood sugar once again. One of the responses to a low level of blood-sugar is a subjective sense of hunger, and appetite may be increased by this means in patients who have lost interest in food; also, the end of the procedure, perhaps because it closes with a needed meal, is often associated with a feeling of relaxation welcome to those who are otherwise constantly beset by anxiety; and lastly, the treatment carries a placebo effect that is enhanced by the care and attention that it is necessary to give to those undergoing it. In one form or another this low-dosage treatment, known as *modified insulin treatment* to distinguish it from the more stormy insulin coma therapy, is still used in most psychiatric units. Its calming effect is now not so sought after, because sedative and tranquillizing drugs can do the job more successfully and with less trouble, but it is useful for increasing appetite, particularly in the illness *anorexia nervosa* that has a distaste for food as its central manifestation; and like the obsolescent 'deep sleep treatment' it is often prescribed as a placebo, particularly to induce a patient to feel that something definite is being done while in fact the doctors are still making up their minds about diagnosis and treatment.

If the insulin dosage given is too great the blood-sugar may fall excessively and in that event certain physiological effects ensue. The defences of the body are mobilized, as might be expected in view of the biological need for glucose, and the patient becomes restless and alarmed, vigorously secreting adrenaline. If the blood-sugar continues to fall, despite the anti-insulin effect of adrenaline, consciousness becomes clouded and if the condition progresses coma and ultimately death occur. The central nervous system loses efficiency rapidly as the blood-sugar falls because it is for all practical purposes totally reliant for fuel on the glucose circulating in the blood and it cannot, unlike most other organs and tissues, metabolize substitutes even for a short period.

The dosages of insulin used in the early years, though moderate enough, were still able to induce coma, if the patient was left for too long unfed, and the physicians administering the treatment had to be on guard for this complication and ready to deal with it by the administration of glucose via a tube. One of the physicians engaged in this work, Sakel, made observations that were to lead to a great change in the psychiatric treatment of his day.

Sakel noted that those patients who became comatose seemed to be the better for the experience when consciousness was restored, and suggested that patients should deliberately be given comas by using larger does of insulin and allowing it longer to take effect. After much trial and error the difficult technique of insulin coma therapy was worked out, and the indications for the treatment were recognized as being confined to the acute schizophrenias. By the beginning of the Second World War this treatment, sometimes combined with electric treatment if concurrent indications for this existed, was in use in most of the mental hospitals of the civilized world.

At the present time, though few psychiatrists believe that we have a completely specific remedy for schizophrenia, few hospitals maintain an insulin unit, and those that do seldom use it to capacity. The story of the rise and fall of this kind of treatment, used in its hey-day on such figures as the dancer Nijinsky, and occupying the most active hours of the doctors and nurses of the majority of hospitals and psychiatric units, is a fascinating one, and one that may not be complete even today.

Certainly, there were plenty of reasons for abandoning insulin coma treatment at the first sign of a simpler remedy of comparable usefulness. It produced a definite rate of mortality, it tied up many nurses and doctors day in and day out and, with an average course of forty to sixty comas, it took many weeks to complete. When electric treatment was introduced in the nineteen-thirties there was a move to stop or reduce the use of insulin coma therapy, until it was found that the indications for the two treatments were different. Many years later, when chlorpromazine was introduced into psychiatric work and found to be effective against schizophrenia, the opportunity of economizing on doctors' and nurses' time without apparent detriment to the patients' progress was widely taken.

Even before the introduction of the major tranquillizers not everybody agreed that insulin coma treatment had any specific value. Those who dissented from the then general opinion agreed that patients often improved during the course of comas, but argued that this benefit depended on a combination of favourable incidentals, such as increased personal attention, team activity, and the dangers shared and overcome, if it was not merely a chance recovery whose spontaneity was disguised by the treatment that was being coincidentally administered. However, insulin coma treatment had been introduced and accepted without a controlled trial of the type described in Chapter 2, and its critics had to accept that it was too late to perform one. The treatment, rightly or wrongly, had acquired a reputation for efficacy and it was therefore no longer possible to set up an experiment in which some of the acute schizophrenics at a hospital received insulin coma treatment while others, randomly selected, did not, lest doing so might deny possible benefit to the patients used as controls.

Restricted by their ethics, the best the disbelievers could do at this time was to compare the respective outcomes in those patients who had received the treatment and those who, for one reason or another, had not. These comparisons were unsatisfactory because there was no way of guaranteeing that the two groups compared were originally alike; often patients who did not receive insulin coma treatment were denied it because it was felt that treated or untreated their chances of improvement were very small, so that it was not surprising that when this kind of comparison was made the coma-treated groups turned out to have done better. However, the publication and verbal dissemination of figures and arguments failing to support insulin coma treatment had little effect on the therapeutic policies of the psychiatrists of the thirties and forties. Probably the main reason why those who doubted if insulin coma therapy accomplished anything did not obtain a hearing was that psychiatrists were unwilling to be robbed of their only active method of combating the main disease of their speciality. Certainly, it was not until tranquillizers were well established, with their effects not only on the realm of treatment but on the rigour and degree of refinement of therapeutic trials, that the first 'blind' comparison was done.

This trial was carried out by B. Ackner and his associates and remains an object lesson. It set out to satisfy the following criteria:

The patients selected should all have undoubted schizophrenia and be such that all experienced psychiatrists would regard as good subjects for the [insulin coma] treatment. The patients should thus all have a clearly defined onset of symptoms of under one year's duration and should not have had an insidious onset or a marked abnormal personality.

The age range should be such as to exclude the menopausal and adolescent psychoses, which may have a different prognosis.

To avoid including those with a tendency to rapid remission, patients should not be accepted until a few weeks after their admission.

Those undertaking the insulin therapy should not be responsible for the selection, diagnosis, and subsequent assessment of the patients.

The schizophrenic group so selected should be divided into diagnostic sub-types because these are usually believed to differ in their outcome, and the sub-types should be separately randomized into treatment and control groups. Both these groups should be treated contemporaneously under the care of the same doctors and nurses. They should be treated in the same ward; and, except for the actual administration of insulin, the controls should receive treatment which in all other respects is comparable to that given to the insulin group.

Those originally responsible for selecting the patients should assess results without any knowledge of the treatment received by the patients. This assessment should be made in accordance with previously agreed and defined criteria, and it should be made at suitable intervals after the end of treatment.

The authors reported in 1957 that twenty-five matched pairs had been treated, the treatment group with insulin comas and the controls with deep sleep or coma induced by barbiturates and terminated by dextroamphetamine: in this way all patients could be treated virtually alike, all became unconscious, all were woken by fluids (sugar or dextroamphetamine), and all participated in the beneficial group effort of the busy insulin centres. Follow-up showed that 40 per cent of both groups recovered fully, and thereafter that, though coma treatment of one kind or another might be of benefit to acute schizophrenics, 'the results suggest that insulin is not the specific therapeutic agent'. A three-year follow up reported later showed no evidence of any superiority of the remissions undergone by the insulin-treated group; indeed, if anything, the insulin-treated patients did worse in later years than the control group.

Trials of this kind are designed to be conclusive; they are meant to determine once and for all whether a treatment possesses real advantages or whether it does not. Yet nowadays though the number of insulin coma units is certainly reduced, the treatment is still used by physicians whose views command respect. That they still believe in the treatment when careful trials have shown it to be of no special worth means that they must base their ideas on vivid personal experience. For this reason it is interesting to recall the way in which patients reacted to insulin coma therapy, to see if it bore the stigmata of a useless treatment.

It was a commonplace that until patients were established on the correct dosage of insulin and deep comas were under way, they were unlikely to improve, though from their point of view their treatments did not differ from those received by their fellows, and any placebo effect was shared by all. Often, however, once the comas were being achieved regularly, improvement was rapid and, some would say, predictable.

The care and management of patients in the insulin coma unit was one of the most exacting of the duties in a psychiatric hospital; the duty was not an unpopular one, however, because of the chance it gave of making contact with patients who were otherwise rendered inaccessible by delusions, pre-occupation with insistent hallucinatory voices, or simply schizophrenic withdrawal. This chance of contact arose when, immediately after the coma, a patient would become lucid and free from symptoms for a few minutes at a time; he might be able to discuss his symptoms, their abnormality, his relief at their departure, and his hopes and plans, only to revert, as the conversation went on, to the world of voices, fancies, and frag-mentation, with the psychiatrist impotently standing by. Each day, in a favourable case, the period of lucidity would lengthen; if with such a patient the course of comas had to be temporarily abandoned because of some chance physical illness, the progress would cease, and might be replaced by retrogression, until therapy was resumed. Many psychiatrists, remembering ex-amples of patients who improved in this steady and solid way, find it hard to believe that they were not watching an effective treatment at work.

As always, psychiatrists are willing to use any so-called remedy if it is the only one available. Insulin coma treatment was stopped at many hospitals because the tranquillizers gave remission-rates that were if anything even more favourable; but for the proportion of acute schizophrenics who do not respond to any of the modern tranquillizers there is little but the older treatments to offer. Fewer may fail to respond to tranquillizers than failed to respond to insulin coma treatment, but there is no theoretical or practical reason for supposing that those who fail with tranquillizers are the very patients who would not have progressed with insulin coma therapy. For these the situation is no gloomier after tranquillizers have failed than the one that faced their forerunners in the nineteen-twenties – unless insulin is tried.

THEORETICAL IMPLICATIONS

Apart from their clinical uses, electric treatment and insulin coma treatment are of great theoretical interest, as any therapies useful in diseases of unknown cause must be.

The epileptic fit itself is a fascinating phenomenon. It is something that is potentially possible in us all. Some of the epileptics who occasionally suffer this paroxysm may be thought of as different from the rest of us not because they have fits but because it is necessary for them to have them; that is to say, that the fit may be an adaptive or protective mechanism of some kind. It is probable that the fit, which is the outward sign of a series of rhythmic synchronous electrically mediated discharges in the brain, is a stereotyped response to certain untoward events in nervous activity, and that the consequence of the fit is that these untoward events and neuronal activities are temporarily extinguished.

If an epileptic patient is monitored on the electro-encephalogram (E.E.G.) during a period that includes a paroxysm, this is seen to be preceded on the record by an increasing series of abnormal electrical discharges and to be followed, once the high-voltage records of the convulsion itself die away, by a period of total absence of cortical activity, represented on the electro-encephalographic tracing by straight lines – so-called electro-encephalographic 'silence'. When electrical activity is resumed over the next minute or two the normal rhythm of the E.E.G. waves re-emerges, but the pathological electrical discharges that preceded the fit do not. It is postulated, by such electro-encephalographic experts as Henri Gastaut, that the fit is the outward expression of the functioning of a massive suppressor mechanism. Such a mechanism is necessary to a computor of the complexity of the brain, so that even if there were no evidence of its existence this would have to be assumed.

Norbert Wiener, the virtual founder of the science of cybernetics, noted that where circular processes, starting by some chance, develop progressively in complex computers this functional fault may be corrected either by clearing the computer of all information (i.e. by switching it off) or by subjecting all parts of the device to a large electrical discharge to interrupt the circuitings. The purpose of the fit, if this is regarded as a method of subjecting the neuronal circuits to an unusually large and repetitive series of discharges, becomes more comprehensible with this analogy. In a metaphorical way the tendency of electric treatment to remove most easily the more recently developed symptoms and to wipe out newly acquired memory traces (often supposed to be laid down initially in the form of dynamic circuitings) is explained. But also certain consequences seem to follow that may have possible therapeutic applications.

It will be remembered that some epileptic patients have premonitory electrical activity that is associated with undesirable psychological symptoms; of these patients it may be said that the sooner the fit occurs the better, and in certain instances, where the fit is preceded by days of mounting irritability or depression, electric treatment has been used empirically to abort the abnormal mood. An analogy may now be drawn between banishing pre-epileptic mood-change, and elevating the mood of the patient in endogenous depression. It is possible that the mood-change of classical depressive illnesses is the consequence of abnormal electrical activity, albeit too subtle for this to be discerned on the electro-encephalographic record, and that it is this that electrically induced fits remove. Before considering this further, the contribution of insulin coma treatment to the argument must be introduced.

In the production of coma after the injection of insulin the reduction of circulating glucose is all-important. The brain relies entirely on this substance for normal functioning, and the effect of depriving the neurones of glucose is first to prevent them from discharging in the normal manner – which leads to altered levels of consciousness – and later to prevent them from living – which is one of the hazards of the treatment. In deep coma, cerebral oxygen consumption, reflecting the overall rate of metabolism in the brain, is reduced and coordinated activity is stopped. When the patient comes round he may show (and if the coma was dangerously deep is specially likely to show) for a time no sign of the schizophrenic symptoms that he displayed earlier in the day; it may be that, as electrically induced fits have been described as parallel to Norbert Wiener's method of clearing a malfunctioning computer by disseminating a large electrical discharge, so insulin coma treatment may correspond to his alternative suggestion – that of switching it off.

These computer-analogies may be superficially feasible; they

are also tenuous and unreliable. Nevertheless they, or speculations like them, have been translated into practical attempts to
extend the range and variety of physical treatments. Development in this field is hampered by one main fact: it is difficult to
reduce the capacity of the neurone to maintain its usual discharging, whether this be abnormal or normal, without also
reducing its capacity to maintain its own cellular integrity. Any
method used that deprives the cell of an essential nutriment
such as oxygen must, in the normal course of events, damage
the neurone. It was on this that early attempts to treat schizophrenics by getting them to breathe pure nitrogen for brief
periods foundered.

There are, however, two possible ways round this dilemma.
The first involves the use of low-temperature anaesthesia; the
second, exploitation of the probability that the neurone uses a
different method of metabolism for discharging from the one it
uses for self-maintenance.

The inability of the brain to withstand prolonged oxygen
lack was a problem in surgery, particularly cardiac and brain
surgery, until advances in anaesthetic techniques overcame this.
At normal temperatures, even when anaesthetized, the brain
uses large quantities of oxygen. If its temperature is reduced the
rate at which molecular activity goes on drops dramatically and
at temperatures that are, though abnormally low, still well above
freezing-point, activity seems to cease altogether. At this stage,
the blood supply to a part may be totally cut off for long periods,
while surgeons replace an artery or refashion the heart, because
no nutriments are needed. Obviously the use of low-temperature
anaesthesia provided a method whereby the brain's functioning
could be stopped without hazarding the life of the individual
neurones, and it was not long before the method was tried. In
the event, it proved impossible to produce low temperatures
with adequate safety (for an experimental technique), and the
negative results at these temperatures did not justify continuing
the trial. It is probable that further efforts will be made to use
low-temperature anaesthesia when the anaesthetic techniques
improve, but at present this research avenue is blocked.

The probability that the neurone has a special metabolism of function, differing from the metabolism taking place within the cell for purposes of maintenance and survival, offers hope of future control of both normal and abnormal functioning. It is likely that certain drugs, such as those used in anaesthesia, affect both the metabolism of function and that of self-maintenance, but do so in a way that causes neuronal discharges to cease long before the cells' vitality is threatened. It may be that the tranquillizing drugs work in a similar fashion, though they, in common with anaesthetics, are used because experience has shown their usefulness and not because any theory of neuronal metabolism indicated that they might be effective. When knowledge of the metabolism of neurones increases, some practical therapeutic developments may follow in the shape of suppression of neuronal function by a chemical agent; in this event pharmacological and physical treatment, which already show some parallelism in their indications and effects, will be combined.

4   Neurosurgical Advances

At one time the investigators of the central nervous system hoped and expected that the experience of anatomists and physiologists who had studied other parts of the body would be repeated, and that they would be able eventually to allocate a certain function to each part of the brain and in particular to each part of the cerebral cortex. In the event, though some cortical areas have been found to have strictly defined functions, such as the areas serving the senses, experimental evidence now indicates that most of the functional units that must exist in the brain are not disposed in an orderly and discrete manner. Most of these units are widespread, and intermingled anatomically with other differently operating units, while the greater part of man's uniquely developed cerebral cortex is probably used in a rotating fashion, i.e. a cell-group becomes available in one of the cortical pools when its last task is finished, rather than being reserved only for certain types of task.

With the lost hopes of cerebral localization went the hopes that neurosurgery could ever be of great importance in the treatment of psychiatric patients as a whole: for if a certain functional unit is overacting in the brain and thereby producing symptoms, its destruction by surgery is liable to be (and in practice is) associated with damage to other units at the same time.

Neurosurgery in psychiatric patients is essentially a mutilating procedure, since the healing that takes place after the operation is confined to the non-nervous tissue, and no regeneration of neurones takes place. Its potentialities are therefore limited, and for this reason, this chapter will look backwards rather than forwards though the prospects for psychosurgery, as it is sometimes called, will be mentioned at the end.

The story of psychosurgery is mostly that of the rise and fall of the operation of prefrontal leucotomy (lobotomy), and most of the pitfalls and hazards of surgical intervention in psychiatric patients can be illustrated by the history of this procedure.

Clinical experience with subjects with brain injuries, such as those who had sustained and survived penetrating wounds of the skull, showed that damage to the frontal lobes of the brain produced a change of personality rather than an intellectual deficit. The patient typically displayed a cheerful fecklessness and freedom from care associated with some deficiency in foresight, but his memory and intelligence were not necessarily simultaneously impaired, except for fall-off occurring as a result of inattention and carelessness. Corresponding evidence of the effects of frontal-lobe damage was provided by patients with cerebral syphilis (G.P.I.), a condition that often produced a mental state of insouciance and showed, at post-mortem, a preponderance of damage in the frontal area. Since many psychiatric patients suffer from an inability to achieve cheerful relaxation of any kind, it is not surprising that this crude clinical knowledge, backed as it was by extensive animal experiments, was ultimately exploited by surgeons interested in the central nervous system. The earliest recorded example of surgical intervention along logical lines took place in the nineteenth century, but it was not until shortly before the Second World War that W. Freeman and J. W. Watts were bold enough to undertake a large series of operations. This trial took place in the United States and later the operation was adopted by Great Britain and many other countries, with a consequent extension of research and development.

The original operations, however they were done, and whatever instrument, blunt or sharp, was used to interrupt the pathways, isolated a large proportion of the frontal lobes from the main central relay nucleus, the thalamus. At first the operations caused damage that was too extensive and they were largely used, as are so many new procedures in the experimental stage, on chronic schizophrenics who are not now thought to be ideal recipients of this operation. The results reflected these serious flaws: too many patients became totally inert and unresponsive; some died at once; others died some months later from obscure disturbances of control function exerted by the cortical areas involved; some patients improved but many did not, and a few became worse.

Opposition to the operation, already strong, became stronger, but the surgeons and the psychiatrists who collaborated with them carried on. In 1950 the operation was banned in the U.S.S.R., while at the same time enthusiastic reports of undeniable successes started to be heard from widely separated psychiatric centres. There was something to be said on both sides but while the debate continued the evidence on which participants were basing their arguments altered.

Because all the members of the teams of doctors concerned in leucotomizing patients were acutely aware of the hazards and the singularly responsible nature of the step taken when the operation was advised, the patients who did undergo the operation were subjected to intense scrutiny during the postoperative months and years. Painstaking follow-up assessments of large numbers of patients enabled physical and psychiatric complications of the surgical intervention to be weighed and, even more important, allowed the indications for the operation to be precisely set out.

The surgical complications – death, excessive disruption due to local haemorrhage, and post-operative epilepsy – were those of any brain operation. Any decrease in their incidence would have had to come from a general advance in brain-surgery and these complications had to be accepted as an inherent part of the risk of undergoing leucotomy.

The psychological complications, on the other hand, were peculiar to this operation. Though leucotomy was done on the basis of some small knowledge of the functions of the frontal lobe, it was not until the operation had been used many hundreds of times that these functions became fully appreciated. The frontal lobes seem to be concerned with the imposition, on a more primitive pattern of behaviour, of restraint and of simultaneous weighing of immediate and distant considerations, social consciousness, and the dictates of conscience. They also subserve in some way the functions that include drive, initiative, and spontaneity.

The psychological complications of excessive frontal-lobe damage may therefore be disastrous. Loss of restraint of a marginal kind might not matter if the patient was not restraining himself markedly before the operation was done. If, on the other hand, he had for years been tolerating, with difficulty and the exercise of much self-control, the irritation of a nagging and unrewarding wife, the post-operative release of rancour might be not only startling to all involved but seem to them relatively ill-deserved; many families of leucotomized patients must have been surprised at the freedom with which patients would speak of old grudges or slights, and have found this difficult to bear; with convalescent patients dependent on their families for much of the rehabilitation and support that is a prerequisite of full success, this possible loss of goodwill was hazardous.

After the operation, also, patients were found to be more attentive to stimuli that offered immediate gratification; patients commonly put on weight, seeming to eat without regard to the price to be paid later in obesity; they spoke on impulse and in a way that was more often appropriate to remarks that immediately preceded theirs rather than the general tenor of the conversation; their disposition to focus attention on immediate considerations made them plan less well, even when the other psychological requirements for good planning were available to them. The reduction in social consciousness made patients less aware of the rights of others, and their weakened consciences sometimes converted this egotism into a callous ruthlessness seemingly foreign to the patient's personality before the operation. On top of all these attitudes and actions there was sometimes laid a grey pall of mental inertia: the patients were generally less able to create, to foresee, to speculate seriously, and to indulge spontaneously in the exploratory and questing manifestations of what is called drive.

On the information about its psychological ill-effects alone it was possible to decide that some patients were unsuitable for the operation because of pre-existing personality attributes which would make the operation unlikely to produce a beneficial overall result. Regardless of the illness and its symptoms, no patient who had shown a pattern of aggression or lack of inhibition, or who had only precariously prevented himself from indulging antisocial desires; no feckless, selfish, or socially irresponsible person; and no patient whose past contained evidence of a serious lack of self-sufficiency and drive could be recommended for the operation without serious misgivings; for it could be confidently supposed that if these failings were great enough to occasion remark or concern before a standard leucotomy they would, in a proportion of patients, be too gross afterwards to allow the patient to make a social recovery.

When the patients were followed up they were found to be divisible into many categories and sub-categories of response. Some might be outwardly improved but deny that they experienced less anguish. Others might hear hallucinatory voices less loudly but resist their antisocial commands with diminished perseverance and thus appear from the outside to be more disturbed or unpredictable. A patient whose series of suicidal attempts tipped the scales in favour of operation might show no desire to end his life after a leucotomy but cease, for the first time, to be gainfully employed. Most of the social failures were those in whom psychological ill-effects enhanced pre-existing flaws, and from these the indications against the use of this operation were determined. What remained to be pinpointed were the factors that could be used to predict positive gain from the operation, and when the results were analysed these were found to be distinct from and in many cases totally independent of the patients' diagnoses.

It transpired that the patients who improved were principally those who suffered such symptoms as severe anxiety, tension, fearful remorse, and recurrent and repetitive thoughts of an actively unpleasant or unwelcome nature – who suffered, in a phrase, 'tortured self-concern'. Certain illnesses, such as obsessive-compulsive neurosis, were liable to impose symptoms of this kind on the patient; others, such as chronic schizophrenia, less likely. The important finding was that it was the symptom rather than the illness that the treatment removed; where the symptom virtually constituted the manifestations of the illness the operation succeeded, but where the tension and anguish comprised little of the symptomatology the most notable result of operating might be the infliction of unwelcome psychological side-effects.

Sobered by the surgical and psychological complications and guided by the knowledge of factors that could be used to make successes more frequent, psychiatrists requested and obtained modifications of the original (standard) operation and selected their patients for the operation on a more informed basis. During the nineteen-fifties the standard operation became less and less popular and leucotomies were more frequently of a minor and less traumatic type. Contrary to expectations the modified leucotomies produced reductions in symptoms as marked as those which followed the more radical early operations, and they happily did so with minimal or undiscernible personality change.

By this time, however, the influence of the unsuccessful patients was making itself felt: no one working in mental hospitals could fail to be affected by the daily sight of cabbage-like patients, emotionally bleached and intellectually inert, and it was these patients who contributed more to the image of the operation than the early patients who became well and left the hospital or the later patients who improved after the modified procedure. Thus the operation fell into disrepute with many who had advocated it, at a time when its defects were being largely eradicated.

Other factors contributed to the reduction in the numbers of leucotomies done. The quality of the results obtained depended very greatly on the standards of post-operative care and the rehabilitation measures that were undertaken, and these essentially social measures formed part of a general revival of interest in the therapeutic milieu, which in turn was a reflection of the increased optimism in psychiatry now that radical treatments were available. Such social measures of activation and group participation, with regeneration of personal pride in cleanliness, were found to produce results in noisy and deteriorated patients that often made the use of the operation unnecessary. By the mid nineteen-fifties, the phenothiazine drugs were bringing about improvement in the chronic patients of mental hospitals, and replenishing the optimism of the medical and nursing staffs: these drugs were most effective when used on acute patients but they led to a crop of startling improvements even from the unpromising soil of the back wards of old mental hospitals, and reinforced the psychiatrists' awareness that chronically ill patients were not necessarily incurable. No one could be certain what the next year might bring, and psychiatrists hesitated to leucotomize, even when the indications were substantial and clear, lest a new drug made the operation obsolete for the chronic schizophrenic.

Later in the nineteen-fifties the anti-depressive drugs came into use, and the chronically depressed patient who might otherwise have been recommended as suitable for leucotomy was offered another therapeutic chance: though the anti-depressive drugs work poorly on chronic depressions, they promise further improvement, and make psychiatrists hesitate to suggest operation. The obsessive-compulsive patient, harassed by the need to carry out purposeless rituals and torn between resistance to the impulses and the wish to reduce unbearable tension, is one of those in whom a good result may be most confidently predicted, but even this type of patient may respond to some of the newer drugs (if early reports are to be trusted) and the surveys of series of cases show that the outlook for the untreated, once thought very poor, is in the long term quite hopeful – facts that combine to make psychiatrists hesitate to propose operation even to this group of patients.

Nowadays a few hundred patients in any one year, carefully selected and reviewed, undergo one of the modified forms of leucotomy. The operation deals only with symptoms, whereas the new drug treatments often deal with actual diseases: as more specific treatments are discovered, or as more reliable variants of existing specific treatments are developed, the number of diagnoses appended to the patients who are leucotomized will fall, to the relief not only of those who oppose the operation but of those who recommend and perform it. But prefrontal leucotomy has conferred great benefits in its time: it cured a few, relieved many, enabled drugs to effect improvement which before operation had produced negligible effect, and had as its principal target the symptom of anguish. As long as extremes of discomfort continue to beset patients indications for its occasional use may arise.

Epileptic fits occur when the deep nuclei of the brain initiate and maintain a series of massive discharges. To the observer the epileptic subject appears struck down, perhaps with a cry; the muscles go into a prolonged spasm (the tonic phase) on which is imposed, after a few seconds, a rhythmic pattern of contractions of all the muscles of the body (the clonic phase). The frequency and excursion of these contractions gradually lessen, and the patient starts to breathe stertorously. Consciousness, which is lost at the start, returns after a few minutes and unless the patient falls asleep he can go about his business a short while later. Fits of this kind are a common cause of falls in the street and, as the use of electric treatment has shown, they can be induced in anyone if the disrupting stimulus is great enough.

Patients who suffer from epileptic fits fall generally into two overlapping classes. There are those who have fits, so it seems, because their liability to react in this way is constitutionally great – who have seizures without any obvious cause being found; and there are the patients whose epilepsy follows the development of some scar, usually in the cerebral cortex, that leads to abnormal electric discharges which seem to induce epileptic fits in the patient. The first group may be called idiopathic and the second symptomatic epilepsies. It is also convenient to call the epilepsy of the first group 'generalized' and that of the second, symptomatic group 'partial', because of their different electro-encephalographic and clinical signs.

Patients suffering from idiopathic epilepsy (that is, epilepsy of unknown cause) have seizures that come on suddenly and are not associated with any other abnormality. The electro-encephalogram confirms the clinical expectation by showing that the electric discharges start suddenly and symmetrically; and if the brain of such a patient is examined no pathological features are found except such as may be accounted for by the occurrence of frequent fits. This type of epileptic often has a family history of seizures, and seldom has any item in his past history, such as birth trauma or severe head injury, that might plausibly account for the development of fits. In a broad sense, this type of idiopathic generalized epilepsy does not constitute an illness. The patients would be well advised to modify their lives somewhat, avoiding, for example, trades like steeplejack and bus driver – though not all of them do; and they may, because of their own sensitivity, avoid social contacts lest they embarrass their friends or themselves by having a fit in company, overrating the alarm fits cause. But this type of patient does not turn up at psychiatric clinics and indeed would not have to see a doctor at all were it not necessary to check from time to time that he is suitably adjusted to and displaying no severe side-effect of his anti-epileptic medication. No special personality can be attached to these patients, nor any serious predisposition to other disease.

Partial epilepsy, symptomatic of some localized lesion in the brain, is, despite the great similarity of the seizure itself, very different in many of its characteristics and particularly in its consequences for the personality and the patient's psychiatric state. Here, characteristically the seizure is heralded by an aura – truly, part of the fit itself – when the area of the cortex which contains the epileptogenic focus, whether this be scar-tissue or tumour, starts discharging abnormally and a slow progression of high-voltage electrical activity spreads from the affected area to neighbouring parts of the brain. This electrical activity becomes more widespread, and may ultimately trigger off a *grand mal* convulsion – the major fit. But until it does so consciousness, though it may be altered or clouded, is not entirely lost and the patient experiences strange sensations (arising from the activation of sensory cortex) or undertakes purposeless movements (if cortex concerned with motor activities is affected). The aura depends for its nature on the area containing the epileptogenic focus: if this lies in the visual cortex, flashes of light are seen; if in the motor cortex, the subject feels twitchings of muscle groups: the site of the lesion can be determined with considerable accuracy and reliability by simply listening to the patient's story. In one special case, the only one of major psychiatric concern, the patient experiences complex psychic phenomena, and his activities may be strange, bizarre, and frightening: also, between seizures, the patient may display a disordered personality, particularly one of aggressive resentfulness, or overt psychiatric illness ranging from psychoneurosis to psychosis. In these instances the epileptogenic focus is usually to be found in one or both temporal lobes, and the condition is called temporal-lobe epilepsy or, because of the outward manifestations, psychomotor epilepsy.

The cerebrum, the large mass of white and grey matter that constitutes the principal distinguishing feature of the human brain, is divided by deep fissures into several pairs of lobes. The temporal lobes, underlying the temples, are concerned with the function of hearing and the development of emotional states; they are also concerned in some way with memory and the process of remembering, and have close functional and anatomical relationships with a near-by area, which subserves smell and takes part in the control of emotional responses.

It is not surprising that a spreading electric discharge, involving an increasing area of this cortical felt, should produce complicated psychological manifestations, since unless and until the discharge becomes gross enough to precipitate a full-scale convulsion, consciousness is largely retained. As the aura starts, the patient may experience crude hallucinations of smell and taste, or of sensations arising from the alimentary canal or of hearing. More elaborate hallucinations, depending on the effects of discharges in the areas serving memory, may recall scenes or sounds of long ago or lie behind the phenomena of panoramic memory and dreamy states; these symptoms, essentially those of altered memory and consciousness, shade off into the common (i.e. normal) anomalies of *déjà vu* (the sensation of having seen what one is looking at at some time in the past, though a previous visit cannot have occurred) and *jamais vu* (the feeling that a scene that should be familiar is in some fashion novel), both of which may occur with great intensity in temporal-lobe attacks. Also associated with the aura are emotional states, usually autonomous but sometimes appropriate in quality to some situational stimulus, and which include fear, depression, and attacks of rage. Temporal-lobe epileptics constitute about 25 per cent of all epileptics seen by neurologists in outpatient departments, but more than 75 per cent of the epileptic patients found in specialized epileptic colonies or mental hospitals have temporal-lobe foci. The high proportion among institutionalized epileptics is an indication of the extent to which the fits or the interseizure behaviour patterns of these patients are antisocial or personally distressing.

Like other types of epilepsy, the temporal-lobe attacks can be made less frequent by anti-epileptic medication, but temporal-lobe epilepsy is unusually difficult to control in this way and, perhaps because of the normalizing effect which a seizure has on this type of epileptic, a pharmacologically induced reduction in seizure-rate can lead to a sharp worsening of the patient's psychiatric condition: one patient who underwent severe depression and agitation during the days before his fit learnt to stop his anti-epileptic medication abruptly, resuming it on regaining both consciousness and ease of mind after the inevitable fit had taken place. Certain patients are unresponsive to all available drugs and régimes: their fits continue intractably despite attempts to find an effective combination of anti-epileptic medications, and it proves impossible to reduce the severity of the illness by ameliorating the psychological stresses that so commonly precipitate psychomotor attacks.

Some of these patients may be successfully operated upon, but certain precautions in selection must be taken if catastrophe is to be avoided. The indications for operation are fairly clear – if the fits are severe, particularly if they are associated with psychiatric abnormality, or if they are worsening, the downhill course suggesting the presence of an expanding mass of tumour tissue. However, the operation consists of the removal of the temporal lobe, and the consequences of the loss of this lobe will, under certain circumstances, be disastrous.

If the temporal lobe of a normal person is removed, say, after its disorganization by a penetrating missile, the effects are usually negligible: temporal lobectomy on the non-dominant side (the right in right-handed persons) makes no difference, and on the dominant side causes only a reduction in the ability to learn items that are heard (as distinct from seen or felt). The temporal lobes act in concert and there is much duplication of function so that the removal of one simply makes the functioning of the other more crucial. In temporal-lobe epilepsy, however, the second lobe may be unable to support the load thrown upon it by removal of the first. If one diseased temporal lobe is removed and the other turns out to be ineffectual the patient becomes totally unable to memorize anything at all, displaying a type of memory defect never otherwise seen except in rare cases of encephalitis and vitamin deficiency, and becoming totally unable to live a normal life. All too frequently the insult that causes temporal-lobe scarring, whatever it may be, does so on both sides. If, however, the lobe that is less affected is still capable of performing most of its functions, it may do so more efficiently after amputation of the opposite lobe because it is made free of the disorganizing impulses that emanated from its counterpart.

The selection of the patients suitable for operation is not easy. As the indications and hazards have become clearer, mainly through successes and failures during the late nineteen-fifties, the results have improved. Not only is the primary aim of the operation – control of seizures – often attained, but even when this is not complete, improvements in psychiatric states are regularly seen; the psychological symptoms do not show the paradoxical worsening sometimes found after drug-induced seizure control. Immediately after the operation (removal of the anterior five centimetres of the temporal lobe) the patient may develop an acute psychotic state, but this responds readily to the usual remedies. Generally psychological improvement continues for some time after operation. About a quarter of the patients show full psychiatric recovery, and another quarter improve considerably – high proportions in view of the incidental nature of the psychiatric disability when operation is being considered.

The mortality from the operation is about one per cent, a price that is well worth paying for the relief of drug-resistant severe epilepsy, but too high to make the operation in its present form suitable for use on purely psychiatric grounds. The increased interest taken in temporal-lobe epilepsy since the advent of specific operative treatment has enabled psychiatrists to refine considerably their ideas on the subject.

The histories of patients show that they often have episodic attacks of mood-change – often depression or anxiety, but sometimes dangerous aggression. They may also have psychotic episodes of greater or lesser length, and personality changes that seem permanent. Any or all of these psychological changes may take place before any fits have occurred, so it follows that if a patient displays any of these phenomena, even without fits, the diagnosis may be one of temporal-lobe epilepsy and the management of his depression or aggression will then have to be neither purely anti-depressive nor punitive, temporarily effective though these measures may be, but anti-epileptic. With the surgical treatment of temporal lobectomy, as with pre-frontal leucotomy, secondary diagnostic and therapeutic gains for psychiatry have followed the use of the operation.

THE SURGICAL TREATMENT OF PARKINSONISM

Parkinsonism is a neurological condition involving a coarse tremor, particularly of the hands, a fixed facial expression and an awkward gait. It may occur as a late sequel of encephalitis lethargica (so-called sleepy sickness), which constituted an epidemic after the First World War, or from arteriosclerotic changes in the vessels supplying the deep extrapyramidal nuclei of the brain, or simply because of unexplained degeneration of these nuclei. Its psychological accompaniments are few, though as usual they are becoming more appreciated as the use of specific and successful treatments call for a closer look at the patients: often the patients show depression, and though this would be easy to account for in terms of a natural emotional response to the disabling nature and downhill course of the illness, it is sometimes found to have preceded by months or years the development of neurological symptoms. They may also complain of a particular difficulty with speech – a blocking of the process of formulation of sentences that causes them to stop suddenly and lose the thread of their conversations: this blocking is different in quality from that seen in schizophrenia, but the patients' descriptions of it call those of the schizophrenics to mind.

As medical psychologists, psychiatrists are interested in the consequences of any brain injury, if only for the light it may throw on the function of the part affected. Usually brain operations are done to save life, and the cost in loss of function may be high. If an operation were not mutilating, but produced an immediate improvement of function, psychiatric interest would be mobilized by the possibility of exploiting the change in psychiatric treatment, as was done with prefrontal leucotomy. Few operations done on the brain offer anything so hopeful, and even the highly effective operation for parkinsonism might not be of great immediate interest if it were not for the status of parkinsonism as a side-effect of drugs used in schizophrenia.

It is a remarkable fact that all the very different chemicals thought to be successful in the treatment of schizophrenia – reserpine and its congeners, the phenothiazines, and haloperidol and similar drugs – consistently produce parkinsonism or other 'extra-pyramidal' side-effects if used in dosages suitable for the treatment of an acute psychotic. It is possible that the production of parkinsonism is in some way important in the suppression or eradication of schizophrenic processes. It is only in the last few years that the development of precise and exacting localizing techniques (stereotaxis) have allowed parkinsonism to be treated surgically with consistent success, but the patients who undergo the operation have been tested and scrutinized pre- and post-operatively to determine the precise psychological changes that have taken place, particularly in the hope of finding out some more about the basic mechanisms of schizophrenic symptomatology. Interestingly, some recent work seems to show that this operation, even if comparatively unsuccessful in dealing with the parkinsonism, produces a marked improvement in the patient's mood.

THE PROSPECTS FOR
PSYCHOSURGERY

In the immediate future there may be a small swing of the pendulum in favour of leucotomy, because the largely beneficial results of discriminating, modified procedures are becoming well known. The old standard operation, which is still occasionally used, will probably be entirely abandoned. The operation, standard or modified, will persist only for as long as other remedies for the illnesses concerned are unavailable. Operations for temporal-lobe epilepsy may be done more frequently as the safety and predictability of the procedure improves, so that it may ultimately be used specifically for the rather uncommon psychoses or gross behaviour disturbances of which temporal-lobe epilepsy is the prime cause. It would be fair to say, however, that unless some remarkable new function of some discrete structure in the brain is found, surgical treatment of psychiatric conditions is very unlikely to be extended. The manner in which it will assist psychiatric work will mainly be in the new knowledge of the function of various parts that will accrue as careful follow-up studies are done on patients who have had these removed at operation. Psychiatrists associated with neurosurgical centres are exploiting for the benefit of fresh generations of patients the observations that may be made on the casualties of the present day.

THE PSYCHIATRIC ASPECTS OF
SEVERE BRAIN DAMAGE

In most instances patients who sustain severe brain damage die fairly shortly afterwards: this is because most strokes take place in the elderly and constitute evidence of severe and widespread arterial disease in the brain, while most large-scale excisions of brain tissue are undertaken for the relief of tumour-symptoms, easing the patients' last months rather than lengthening life, these two conditions – strokes and tumours – being the commonest causes of gross damage. Such patients are in many ways unsuitable subjects for research into the social and psychological effects of the particular damage done, not only because they live too short a time but because the extent of the damage varies and increases as time goes by.

Certain patients sustain strokes, however, who are young and likely to live on for a long period. These patients often bleed from sac-like expansions of their cerebral arteries, called aneurisms, and when they do so are extensively investigated because it is sometimes possible, though risky, to clip off the aneurism at open operation and thus prevent further bleeding. The patient who recovers from this type of haemorrhage and operation is someone whose brain is probably damaged but who is likely, if he has no more aneurisms, to live a long life: the site and extent of the damage is also known with peculiar certainty because of the precise nature of the investigations that can be done on the cerebral arteries. Follow-ups of these patients are being done on a large scale not only to find out the neurological effects in terms of paralysis and degree of recovery, but the effects on intellectual and social function of the loss of individual areas of the brain. In this respect it is unlikely, in view of what we know from general impressions of patients who have had cerebral damage, that any of the consequences will be desirable and therefore of possible use in psychiatric work, but psychiatric skills will enable the difficulties that beset these patients to be more precisely formulated, with consequent improvement and psychological refinement of the treatment and rehabilitatory measures used. To some extent it is to be hoped that knowledge of brain function will also increase, so that this work is part of the effort to construct a working scheme of brain function, the lack of which makes so much of psychiatry a guessing game.

New Methods in
Psychiatric Hospitals

Psychiatric hospitals exist to save life, to comfort or cure, and to provide custody, but the order of priority of these aims has altered over the years.

Two centuries ago lunaticks who survived the acute phase of the illness might be fortunate enough to have dependable relatives or might in rare instances be admitted to Bethlem, then the only asylum, but for the most part they were confined either in poor-law institutions or in private madhouses, or, what might be the worst of all, kept locked up alone in private households. Only exceptionally would they escape treatments that were, with the best intentions, deliberately terrifying or, with good but more practical intentions, meant to weaken. If they fell into the hands of the more unscrupulous keepers of private madhouses, whose practices were one of the scandals of a scandalous age, their liberty might be permanently, because profitably, taken away; and even if their detention lasted only as long as the active illness it was emphasized by humiliating and goading shackles.

At the end of the eighteenth and beginning of the nineteenth centuries some definite movements towards reform started, the origins of which were various and obscure. The British public was easily alarmed by the idea of allowing lunatics to wander abroad, and less troubled, at that time, by the mistreatment of asylum inmates; but as always there was a strong response to tales of the forcible incarceration of the sane without due process of law or any chance of appeal, and if only on these grounds some measure of control was demanded. In France Pinel had shown, by striking off the shackles of his insane patients, that to do so was to cause an immediate improvement in psychological well-being. In England the treatment of George

III, who could not be regarded by his loyal subjects as a typical lunatic but who was, nevertheless, undoubtedly mad for much of his reign, had shown that mental illness was recoverable but that some of the treatments were unpleasant; also that lunacy was compatible with intelligence, godliness, personal bravery, and high birth. Before 1800 Bethlem (Bedlam) Hospital, which had operated in solitary splendour or disgrace, according to who was describing it, since 1377, had been reinforced by three new hospitals including one, The Retreat at York, which was showing what moral treatment, a good diet, and a small community could do for the mentally afflicted.

During the restive days of the French Revolution and the Napoleonic wars that followed some of the reformist zeal in the air was even felt by mental hospitals. The need for in-patient treatment was clear to all and it was generally agreed that treatment, if delayed, would fail to deal with the illness. Many of the ideas of the times were, however, concerned with the liberty of the subject. The English felt that this was their special province and complacently supposed that, because it permitted greater freedom of thought, this liberty was the cause of their allegedly high incidence of madness (in which, then as now, they took a curious collective pride).

Thus although in the early nineteenth century the legislature passed laws encouraging local authorities to build mental hospitals, and in the middle of that century the Government explicitly required that local authorities should undertake this work, at the same time (1845) the Lunatics Act made certification so cumbersome and difficult a procedure as to ensure that it would only be the lot of the deeply disturbed. Mild or early cases would on the whole not be liable to the provisions of the Act and would therefore not be admitted to the new hospitals, which could only take certified patients.

The Victorians were high-minded, bold, and honest. In the years that followed the request that mental hospitals be built these comparatively unproductive buildings were erected by the score. They were sited at the outskirts of the towns, partly because land was cheaper in the country, but also because there the patients could do simple farming tasks which were supposed to be naturally healthy, partly because the air in towns was badly polluted at the height of the industrial revolution and it was felt that in the absence of specific treatment fresh air might help; and because, no doubt, it was thought preferable to isolate the community from the sight and sound of the insane.

The Victorians built them large, and as time went by, larger, not because they thought that big hospitals were ideal (the mid nineteenth century psychiatric opinion about optimum size was about 250 beds) but as a consequence of finding that whatever size a hospital was built it always became overcrowded within a year or two. No doubt they might, in a given instance, have built several small units of 300 beds instead of one of the single unmanageable 1,200-bed mammoths that house most of the country's psychiatric patients, but the large hospitals had compelling administrative economies to offer and at least the excessive centralization practised in such American cities as New York, where most psychiatric patients are to be found in hospitals of more than 5,000 beds, was avoided.

These hospitals were built to last. Their appearance, even when softened by pleasant gardens, is often monstrous, but they are aesthetically no worse than some of the brick churches that moulder in the suburbs of London and the Northern industrial towns: within, amenities and decoration were excellent – given the standards of the time. The builders were aware that the patients came from poor, ill-equipped, and insanitary homes, and planned buildings that were imposing and grand because it was their aim to produce uplift. They knew that the shock of leaving home, be it never so humble, and entering an institution under duress, had to be countered as far as possible despite the increased cost. Thus, at a time when all kind of public and private investment was being undertaken and when the country, by the standards of today, was bitterly poor, a hundred hospitals costing a quarter to half a million pounds each were put up for paupers who could not vote.

These mental hospitals are with us today and indeed, with a handful of exceptions and a few modifications, provide the whole of the psychiatric in-patient services of the country. One is to be found on the outskirts of any large town, and their battlemented water towers ring London like a chain of outmoded fortresses. It is hard to generalize satisfactorily about the treatment that was given at these hospitals before the First World War: probably there was as little brutality as there was hope in most of the hospitals. In some, noble traditions or the chance factor of an optimistic superintendent caused isolated or recurrent waves of activity, followed quickly by reaction. Indeed, the therapists were in an impossible dilemma if they regarded their task in the traditional medical manner – and few of the doctors had any training in psychiatry over and above experience in a mental hospital learning the old ways of dealing with the insane: the ancient remedies of bleeding and purging were abandoned, but there was nothing to take their place.

In retrospect it is possible to single out from the writings of the nineteenth century those pioneers who pointed out that giving liberty, the exchange of trust, and the provision of useful work and gentle example was followed by magnificent results, but so many other measures were also proposed that it must have been hard, at the time, to choose between them. Depressingly, the superintendents (until 1948 the uncrowned kings of the mental hospitals) seem to have ignored the measures that promised some human dignity to their patients and concentrated on the custodial side of their work; at a time when much of their responsibility lay in ensuring that the legal form of detention was beyond any possible question and a good deal of their clinical timetable (e.g. how many ward-rounds per day were done) was decided by statute, they may be forgiven for requiring no more than that the social and occupational measures which were in force did not deteriorate. Certainly, one feels that as long as the public were not prepared to see patients going to mental hospitals unless they were so disordered as to seem to a magistrate unsuitable to be abroad, the mental hospitals could hardly improve.

During the opening years of the twentieth century the psychiatrists resolved this dilemma (whereby patients could not be enticed to present early in the illness unless they knew they could avoid going to a mental hospital) by starting in-patient care outside the mental hospitals. By the time that the first of these 'undesignated' hospitals, the Maudsley, was opened in 1923, the public had a different and more vivid idea of mental illness from First World War veterans with shell-shock. Most of the 'shell-shock' cases are now known to have been hysterical, but many were looked upon with a sympathy that persisted even when, after the war ended, the symptoms disappeared.

Between the wars several general hospitals started to admit psychiatric patients and the psychiatrists on their staffs ran out-patient clinics of a diagnostic kind. The rapid development of out-patient psychiatry during the twenties and thirties depended not only on the provision of a suitable service for a pool of distressed people for whom hitherto there had been nothing to offer unless they became certifiable, but on the influence of Freudian ideas which seemed to offer treatment for the psychoneuroses. Indeed, so long as there were no physical treatments at all, these ideas constituted the only hope for patients whose illnesses could not be relied upon to remit naturally; psychiatrists turned eagerly from the long-standing cases in the mental hospitals to the early and presumably more hopeful subjects they could see at a hospital out-patient department.

By the start of the Second World War most mental hospitals had out-patient services, and out-patient work was done at the teaching hospitals, though it was not necessarily exploited for training purposes. Social workers, particularly psychiatric social workers, were first trained formally during the inter-war years. With their assistance the departments became more efficient and the diagnosing psychiatrist was able to take more factors into account. Thanks mainly to Freud, many of the younger men being attracted to psychiatry were less concerned with the easy life it still allowed and more interested in the intricacies of the workings of the normal as well as the abnormal mind. By the time the Second World War started a larger number of competent and enthusiastic psychiatrists were available than there had ever been before.

Even so, most of the mental hospitals were largely untouched by the new spirit. The physical treatments that reached the mental hospitals between the wars were simply grafted on to the existing institutions and an ex-chairman of the Board of Control, looking back on these institutions, could write:

A visit to a mental hospital in the nineteen-twenties was a depressing experience. Most of the hospitals were drab in the extreme and the patients were sullen and often violent, regarding the nurses as gaolers. They had the atmosphere of the old poor-law institutions which, indeed, in many respects they were.

During the nineteen-thirties patients were at last enabled to enter mental hospitals voluntarily if they wanted to and were capable of expressing their wishes, and the use of electric treatment allowed decisive intervention in many cases of depression and some of schizophrenia.

The time was probably ripe for a full-scale modernization of the old places. Partisans of psychiatry may wring their hands because this was not done, but it is not certain that it should have been: modernization and liberalization, which have since been shown to produce great results, would have been thought long-odds bets at that time, and before the Second World War there were many public health problems of greater importance, such as widespread pulmonary tuberculosis, to which a certain answer (early diagnosis and prompt isolation) was known, and which awaited only public funds and a larger share of trained personnel for their final solution.

The passage of the years had not brought much incidental improvement to the great thousand-bed mental institutions. By maintaining standards in only an absolute way the authorities had allowed them to fall behind the expectations of patients living in average family homes: for the patient from Dickens's London tiled walls, green paint, terrazzo floors, square meals, and water-closets represented something like luxury; for the vocal artisan in a thriving industry before the Second World War, institutional squalor.

Even here, in their failure to maintain in a real way what the Victorians had fashioned, the unknown decision-takers were not entirely devoid of sense: in the middle of the nineteenth century the Victorians could spend their money according to priorities decided by the degree of pitiability of the various human afflictions, because they could treat none of them. But once any of the major illnesses became treatable – and all the principal infectious ones became at least controllable by the turn of the century – it would have been perverse to divert money from the demonstrably brilliant work of the bacteriologists of the time to gloomy and uncertain psychiatric endeavours.

The Second World War provided the catalyst for change. At first sight, it brought disaster to the mental hospitals, for staff and doctors, not all of them willing recruits in the first instance (many male nurses came from depressed industries during the slump), left by the hundred for war-service of one kind or another. Grants of money bought less, and day-to-day repairs had to go by the board. Some of the buildings were taken over for emergency surgical hospitals, leading to increased over-crowding in those that mopped up the patients displaced. What stringent rationing and the assessing of priorities according to the necessities of war and the maintenance of public approval meant to the food and dress of the patients can be imagined.

While the mental hospitals continued to go downhill, accelera-ted by the demands of total war, the usual increase in the application of basic knowledge took place in the field, and many medical advances were made. The Germans introduced the sulphonamides just before the war and during its course the British isolated penicillin, as a consequence of which a horde of new remedies was elaborated or discovered. With the greater pharmacological knowledge available, the medical profession was able, at the end of the war, to open a grand attack on disease. The individual illnesses that were reduced from common events in the lives of the citizens of civilized countries to isolated attacks occurring in the unlucky few (or even to curiosities) are well known: diphtheria and other illnesses, notably polio, responded to mass immunization; tuberculosis to the essentially similar method of reducing the infectious pool of sufferers at large in the community; pneumonia, meningitis, syphilis, gonorrhoea, scarlet fever, typhoid, and others were conquered so rapidly by penicillin and later antibiotics that the number of deaths from infectious diseases in the United Kingdom fell from 28,000 in 1946 to 8,000 ten years later. What is not so well known are the implications of these fantastic advances: essentially, what was eradicated was acute disease – and what was left, was chronic.

When chronic illness started to come under the examination of a public and a profession newly attuned to the expectation of cure, the mental hospitals, as the biggest repositories of the chronically ill, could not escape scrutiny. They were found lacking in many respects, though fortunately a good deal of the blame could be diverted on to the Victorians who laboured to build them.

As always, when giving a general account, some over-simplification is necessary to achieve coherence with brevity. Not all the pre-war hospitals were gloomy and forbidding and not all the hospitals of today are even near to the best that they could be within the existing fabric. But the overall picture before the war or just after it was that mental hospitals were locked, therapeutically nihilistic, cut off from the community, autocratic in their social structure, traumatically uncongenial at a domestic level, and geared to dealing with patients whose families had been finally unable to keep them away from the dreaded asylum. Today, in general, none of this is true. What has happened to cause the changes, and which of the changes caused the patients to improve constitutes the substance of this chapter.

THE CHANGES

Some of the changes are easier to discuss than others and their consequences appear deceptively simple. *Electric treatment* came into use just before the war and promptly reduced the time a depressed patient spent in hospital by 70 per cent. *Insulin treatment* probably benefited, directly or indirectly, the acute schizophrenics who received it, and that too was vigorously practised just before and after the war. But these treatments, though they gave doctors a tool or two, did not greatly reduce the complement of patients whose illnesses became chronic, since deep insulin treatment worked best on those schizophrenics likely to recover spontaneously, while depressive illnesses end of their own accord whether they are treated or not, though they may do so only after a long course. However, even though these pre-war treatments did little to relieve the therapists of the morale-sapping treatment-failures in what were called the back wards, one may conjecture that they allowed some hopefulness to arise among both patients and psychiatrists, unfortunate though the idea of 'shock-treatments' was for an already justifiably cautious clientele. For almost a decade after the war no further therapeutic advances of a classically medical kind were made in psychiatry.

Then, in 1954 and 1955, *tranquillizers* were introduced into psychiatric hospitals on a large scale. The pharmacological effects of these drugs are described in detail elsewhere (Chapter 2); whatever they may have done for individual patients and whether their effects were disease-specific or not, they were associated with two lasting phenomena of enormous importance and interest. First, they brought the chronic patients back into the treatable category – at least in the subjective estimation of psychiatrists who apportioned their time according to the possibility of inducing improvement. Second, the year 1955 saw, for the first time since statistics were kept, a reversal in the direction of the graphs depicting the numbers of patients, notably schizophrenics, in mental hospitals in this and other countries of the world; the number of patients in hospital at the end of 1955 was a few hundreds less than at the end of 1954 after a century of remorseless increases, and it seemed that the main difficulty – the terrible load of numbers – might be eased. This downward trend has continued, taking countries or states as a whole, until the present day; but my defensive apologia for over-simplification does not mean that I propose that these gross figures be accepted without further examination, and reference will be made to them again.

The expansion of *out-patient services* and the frequent presence of psychiatrists in general hospital departments meant that between the wars there was a closing of the gap that had come to separate psychiatry from medicine. The new tenets of psychoanalysis, popular with psychiatrists at the time, were not necessarily accepted or approved by the general practitioners, but often enough acquaintance with the person or reputation of a local psychiatrist convinced the G.P. that he was a sensible and useful man to consult. The public were often willing to go to the local general hospital to see a psychiatrist, particularly if he were described as a nerve specialist or as a doctor interested in psychological matters and if the patient were assured that, though nervous or more sensitive than other patients, he was not 'mental' – all these camouflages tended, with the patient's cooperation, to hide the psychiatrist's connexion with the local mental hospital. Also such members of the community as kept up with the latest speculations were aware of the Freudian and neo-Freudian explanations and treatments and no longer regarded quirks or neurotic maladaptations as matters of which they need feel ashamed, at least in a consulting room.

Even before the war the general physicians at the hospital might refer some of their psychologically disturbed patients to psychiatrists on the staff. This departure was probably dictated partly by the usefulness of electric treatment, before the advent of which the general physician could offer almost as much as the psychiatrist – and do so less alarmingly.

All these factors meant that as the thirties, forties, and fifties went by the average patient presented earlier to the psychiatrist. In so far as early treatment usually produces greater success this was to be applauded at any level. But the principal difference it made was that an increasing proportion of patients – still small by the nineteen-fifties – presented willingly, and willingly came to hospital. Such patients possessed expectations and attitudes that contrasted gratifyingly with those of patients protected for years by well-meaning families and finally brought to hospital only as the result of some terrible crisis that needed compulsory admission and detention.

The early out-patient departments were diagnostic in form. A patient would be seen, a history taken, auxiliary information from relatives obtained, and a diagnostic categorization written in the notes, with recommendations for action appended. As out-patient facilities increased, or patients returned again and again to the department that had time to listen (in the words of the teaching aphorism, 'Don't just do something, stand there') and no moral axe to grind, a psychotherapeutic role was added to the original one. Psychiatrists who worked at mental hospitals (the vast majority in the early days of out-patient work, and still the majority) took to filling a great need by seeing recently discharged patients who were struggling to make their way in a hostile or unfamiliar world, and offering advice and support.

The existence of some after-discharge care meant that patients could be let out of hospital at an earlier stage: it was no longer unfair to the patient to send him out on trial if he could return to hospital as soon as his psychiatrist thought he was faltering, rather than waiting until a general practitioner reluctantly found him too difficult to handle outside a mental hospital. The use of the *voluntary status* (introduced by the Mental Treatment Act of 1930 and now obsolete), whereby a patient could sign himself into a mental hospital by agreeing to abide by the rules and give three days' notice of his intention to leave, increased irregularly and unevenly throughout the thirties and, where it was utilized frequently, led to a metaphorical opening up of the hospital, the voluntary patient feeling less cut off from the outside world and the ex-patient struggling at work less far from the haven of the hospital. This ease of entry and discharge was increased greatly when the Mental Health Act (1959) came into force, since which time the entry to and discharge from hospitals has been mainly along *informal* lines, that is to say with no more documentation than is used in a general surgical or medical ward.

This use of mental hospital facilities in a more casual way was until recently marked only in a few of the more enterprising hospital groups, and it took more than a high turnover of patients with relatively mild illnesses to reconcile a community to the jangling keys and rattling locks of the local mental hospital. Since the advent of the tranquillizing drugs and the simultaneous signs of reduction in the total numbers of patients staying in mental hospitals (about 1955), there has been another great development in mental hospital practice: the wards have steadily been unlocked. If the story of the changes in mental hospitals could be summarized by saying that better treatments and better law led to greater turnover, earlier cases, and consequently better results so that finally the wards could be unlocked, it would all be very simple; but only if the sequence is over-simplified to the point of distortion could this summary be offered. This is because, although the bulk of mental hospitals received the impetus and confidence to open their long-locked doors after they had started using tranquillizers, the pioneers of the *open-door* policy had achieved their successes years before this.

How many years before, if isolated or disregarded experiments are considered, casts a slur on the whole of medical psychology. Tuke of The Retreat at York; Pinel; the lay reformers of the early nineteenth century – all knew that the abolition of restraint made patients better. But for many decades the law, though it protected the sane from being found insane, expected those certified as of unsound mind to be firmly shut away; and the responsibility for any escape was the superintendent's alone so that he, in deciding policy, had more to consider (including his reputation) than the patients' immediate welfare.

It was not until the war years that the first influential liberalization of modern times took place, at Warlingham Park Hospital in 1942. At this hospital, and shortly afterwards at Mapperley and other hospitals, the gradual process of unlocking started. Usually it was one man, the superintendent, who initiated and carried through the reform: the powerful nature of the authority vested in the superintendent, a bar to progress if the superintendent was reactionary or passive, became in the case of the men concerned an immense advantage. The poor upward communication in mental hospitals must have been for once an advantage, since any trend towards unlocking doors produced trepidation and resentment in the minds of the established staff of the hospitals.

The pattern of opening the mental hospital was a fairly constant one: the superintendent and his allies, if he had any, pursued a gradual and cautious policy of advance. Perhaps avoiding any outright statement of ultimate aims, the superintendent persuaded the doctors and nurses of the quietest locked ward that it might be worth while trying to open the doors at some future date. Occasional discussions of the possibility led to the staff agreeing: the understanding that the superintendent was responsible for any consequences was well known and comforting for subordinate staff. Usually or often the opening of the doors led to no dramatic untoward events: no mass escapes took place, though often patients would make tentative trial escapes as if to try out the reality of the opened door; no breakdown in orderly discipline occurred and indeed the patients' relationships with the staff improved (as was only natural, it is easy now to point out).

The psychological preparation of the nursing and medical staff for the opening of the first closed ward might take a year. From then on, however, the key reformer acquired influential support: the nursing staff on the open ward were gratified at the improvements they saw, and the word spread. The opening of the second and immediately subsequent wards took place more quickly, though on each occasion the worries of the staff most closely concerned were repeated while those of the superintendent, which as the main distributor of confidence he could hardly express, grew.

Each ward that was opened meant that patients more closely approximating to the popular conception of the insane were given the chance to escape, and each opening ceremony brought the superintendent closer to the refractory wards, within whose walls the most violent and disturbed psychotics resided. Subordinate staff of these pioneer hospitals gained enthusiasm as they went along; for those of us who worked in hospitals with many locked wards it is not easy to see how the superintendents concerned did not lose theirs, why they did not rest on their oars at the half-way mark and call it a well-spent day. The reason they persisted was not that they suffered some neurotic exaggeration of the normal man's distaste for locked doors or were cranks obsessed with seemingly hopeless idealistic reforms like abolishing child-labour; what made them carry on were the incomprehensible changes that they saw in the clinical status of the patients in the newly opened wards.

Chronic psychotics soon lost interest in escaping, stopped

talking about their delusions and suffered less from hallucinations. What had passed for psychotic behaviour for a hundred years was found really to be the result, not purely of mental illness, but of mental illness in a setting of severe restriction of the social freedom and liberty of the person. Once the doors were open the patients needed less, not more, nursing attention and the nurses expressed relief and satisfaction at the new régime. The discharge figures, for what these are worth as a guide to therapeutic success, showed a rise that antedated that associated with the tranquillizers by several years.

This 'open-door' movement grew in prestige and influence during the fifties, but it was not an easy reform to carry out. Without the cooperation of the medical and nursing staff it could not succeed. Without a convinced and dynamic superintendent the junior staff could not be carried along. It took more than simply throwing keys away to make a hospital as well-run as Mapperley. Patients with freedom needed occupation and training; with social freedom, the opportunity to exercise it in congenial surroundings. Fortunately other developments in mental hospital practice were keeping pace with the new demands made by emancipated patients and, providentially, greater public interest in mental health was driving the Government to spend more freely.

In the earliest days of enlightened mental hospital work, a century and a half ago, it was frequently remarked that interesting and productive occupation was helpful to the patients: in this respect pauper patients were better off than their richer confrères, because the well-to-do were kept from work and suffered correspondingly. During the nineteenth century the larger hospitals provided occupations that were mainly concerned with the maintenance of the hospitals themselves, the capitation grant being low enough to encourage superintendents to use this cheap form of labour. Menial tasks, organized from above, are the lot of many of the world's workers, but do not usually provide the whole of the interest and social contact a man experiences: for the in-patient in a mental hospital work that was repetitive, non-productive, and did not pay provided little therapeutic benefit.

It was not appropriate to leave the decision about the therapeutic application of labour to administratively oriented
medical superintendents who apportioned work according to
the requirements of the organization, although in early days the
patients' labour often meant the difference between a hospital
staying adequate and one sinking gradually to fresh depths.
The specialized work of *occupational therapy* was introduced to
provide purely therapeutic application of the old principles, and
during the years immediately before and after the Second
World War many occupational therapists were trained and
started to work in mental hospitals. At first and until quite
recently they used little equipment and the tasks set were of the
arty-crafty type – rug-making, weaving, and so on. These
fancies were the most suitable at the time, no doubt, and
certainly provided an excuse to extract a proportion of patients
from the usual type of work in order to give individual help and
training on work that produced some kind of end-result and
improved confidence and morale.

The patients most affected by the introduction of occupational
therapy were the acute short-stay group, many of them voluntary patients, and a shortage of occupational therapists (except
at hospitals associated with a training school) meant that
chronic and severely disturbed patients were not exposed to this
helpful influence. After the war one kind of treatment was
discovered that could be applied to some chronically violent
patients – prefrontal leucotomy. The old standard procedure
was then the norm, and was often misused, through inexperi-
ence, producing even in successful instances a post-operative
period of inertia and incontinence. It was soon found that the
patients who did best of any given and fairly homogeneous
group were those whose post-operative rehabilitation was most
extensively planned. Occupational therapists were found to be
important figures at this stage of the treatment and they gained
in experience and reputation by successful participation. Their
later development as members of the therapeutic team is bound
up with the altering roles of the nursing staff and will be returned
to at a later stage.

It is convenient to think of the leucotomy operations as

opening the eyes of mental hospital staff to the potentialities of concentrated rehabilitation and habit-training. Like most of the post-war developments this drive to train the patients was simply an application of principles known to lay officials of a hundred years before: many schizophrenic patients were incontinent in the late nineteen-forties, though in the nineteenth century this was known to be preventable or, if established, simply eradicated. It took successes of their own to convince the staff working in the wards, and some early successes came from the leucotomized patients; in some instances their incontinence yielded to post-operative healing processes rather than training, but in many it was the close contact with the nurses and the greater interest and encouragement that was shown that made their personal habits improve. From training leucotomized psychotics it was only a short step to training psychotics whose brains were intact, but it was not until this was tried on a large scale that the hard work really started.

During the years mainly under review – the forties, fifties, and early sixties of this century – the nursing staff underwent a revolutionary change of role. From neutral watchful guardians, saved from inhumanity only by chance personal qualities that made lotteries of their patients' lives, psychiatric nurses have become part of the therapeutic team. The change became radical only when the importance of the nurse's place in treatment was proved by results. These results came from the use of a method known as *total push*, in which everybody, but particularly nurses, attempted to train the patients out of the bad habits that years of neglect (as it would be called now) had allowed them to develop. Nurses took the patients regularly to the lavatory, encouraged them to dress themselves, trained (retrained) them to eat in a civilized fashion, and so on.

Extra nurses were needed to bring about the rehabilitation of a ward-full of deteriorated patients but, once brought up to scratch, less nurses than before were needed from then on because of the patients' ability to attend to their own basic needs. In the forties and fifties hospitals were still being visited by the old independent supervisory body, the Board of Control.

Members of this board wrote official reports on what they found, and once their eyes were opened to the changes that were taking place in the more advanced hospitals they started to encourage other superintendents to introduce the new reforms in their own hospitals; if their suggestions were ignored it was within their power to write an adverse report on the hospital, so that conservatism became risky instead of safe.

One of the last strongholds of conservatism defended the principle of total segregation of the sexes. In the bad old days of the private madhouses one of the best remembered causes of complaint was the sexual licence of attendants and privileged male inmates, and even had this not been so, Victorian morality and its attenuated equivalent of later years justifiably required that patients be protected from their own perhaps disordered sexual desires and those of others. This sexual separation was recognized as artificial and in some ways anti-therapeutic, but it is easy to sympathize with hospital managements who did not care to end it. Some of the neurosis units built or converted to take voluntary patients for psychotherapy allowed some mixing between patients of different sexes and thus it could be said, by the end of the nineteen-thirties, that non-psychotic patients did not misuse the freedom conferred to any greater extent than the public at large.

Some factors can be singled out that led to superintendents experimenting with mixed social groupings: the excellent, normal behaviour of psychotics at a patients' dance was a well-known feature of such psychiatric hospitals as arranged these affairs, and provided an encouraging piece of evidence; the ease with which occupational therapists managed mixed groups of patients was often striking, mixed because they came to the department instead of being supervised in their own wards; and the methods of 'total push', though they ingrained new habits or resuscitated old, did not lead to spontaneity and aliveness, only to greater manageability – that is to say, the patients, having been pushed so far, ceased to improve, and something further was called for. Once patients (and, necessarily, male and female staff) started to mingle, the mental hospital began to resemble, in some ways, a normal community, and it was this aspect of mental hospital organization that then began to interest the innovators.

As usual, they could do no better than refer to the old authorities to find out how the psychotics reacted to some semblance of normal family life. Better documented and detailed work was available from the immediate past, however, and the credit for modern *therapeutic community* methods in mental hospitals must go mainly to psychiatrists practising group therapy with psychoneurotic and psychopathic in-patients, notably Maxwell Jones. Much of this work proved to be directly transferable to mental hospital wards serving psychotics, but the scope of the changes may be judged if the old and the new systems are described.

In the old mental hospital hierarchy of a generation ago the tasks and responsibilities of the staff were all known from statute or tradition. The medical superintendent gave the orders and took the blame. The psychiatrists dealt with the clinical problems and fell in, in general, with the rulings of the superintendent. The senior nursing staff decided which patients constituted clinical problems, and told the doctors. The junior nursing staff communicated their observations and sometimes their views to the senior nursing staff, but not to the doctors. The patients communicated, for the most part, with nobody, turning inwards from the world.

It will be seen that the situations of the participants in these functional units were psychologically secure: the doctors did what the superintendent said and as their professional knowledge directed, the nurses did what their seniors said, and the patients obeyed anybody who spoke to them. Information flowed almost entirely downwards, and what went upwards was modified and formalized to sustain the *status quo* and its satisfactory image. It was possible for a medical officer, a sister, a nurse, and even a patient to lead a very trouble-free life in an old-fashioned mental hospital.

In a hospital whose wards are run on what is called 'therapeutic community' lines all the obvious professional, staff-patient, and senior–junior demarcations became blurred and indented. Doctors, patients, nurses, occupational therapists, psychologists, ward orderlies and all meet once a day for an hour or so and discuss informally what is happening and why. The sub-group with the greatest store of resentment, the patients, speak critically of everybody, including fellow-patients, nurses, and doctors. The junior nurses, if they feel that the assurances they have received about criticism being welcome and no bar to promotion are true, criticize senior nurses and doctors. The senior nurses criticize the doctors. The doctors, used to telling people what to do in organizations geared to saving their feelings in the interests of intellectual effectiveness, try to guide the discussion without shrinking.

Dr D. V. Martin, Medical Superintendent of Claybury Hospital, described in a recent book, *Adventure in Psychiatry*, the extraordinary bitterness and insecurity that the introduction of ward-community methods initially induced in his medical and nursing staff. Here, again, the system is not used simply because the older ways were undemocratic or archaic or deserving of some similar label but because, if enough time is allowed to elapse (about one year), the group discussions become less destructively critical and acrimonious, less concerned with the state of yesterday's macaroni cheese, and more nearly centred on psychopathology and behaviour. The ward atmosphere alters for the better and the patients improve startlingly. The doctors and nurses, once converted, become enthusiastic and say that they would never return to the old methods. The pendulum has swung so far that today, if a mental hospital plays too custodial a role, its staff morale falls.

From this description it might be thought that discipline, support, and pressures arose in some way from within the group, and indeed in the prototypical methods used with patients whose personalities were disordered it was the self-imposition of rules of conduct and responsibility that contributed to the successes. In mental hospitals serving a psychotic group the similarity is superficial; the groups are directed more closely, as disordered groups must be if helpful orientation is to be maintained, and though the wards may be open the threat implicit in the existence of one or two locked wards is ever-present, so that the real authority of the doctors is camouflaged rather than destroyed.

Community methods within the hospital are concerned with the induction of conformity, to an even greater extent than other group methods or individual psychotherapy, but if it is remembered that the method is palliative, aimed at the social consequences of the illness rather than at the disease itself, the beneficial results are, if anything, even more gratifying.

The aims of the old-fashioned superintendent were humane and sensible, if sometimes seeming short-sighted to those rendered long-sighted by the lenses of retrospect, but they seldom included a serious intention to discharge the majority of his chronic schizophrenics. A generation ago a schizophrenic who had been in hospital for two years stood almost no chance of ever being discharged. But in 1955, when the numbers started to go down, a new aim was provided, associated with the competitiveness that attends the possibility of arithmetical comparisons, and the country was swept by a *vigorous discharge policy*. It was necessary for the physician-superintendent with any progressive pretensions to get his patients out. This discharge policy has led to mixed results and some very indigestible statistics (though some planners have swallowed them whole).

As may be imagined, there are many patients in mental hospitals whose conduct includes no positively remarkable features. A patient may believe that he is Joe Lyons's son and Churchill's nephew without constantly finding it necessary to remind others of his antecedents, about which, indeed, the patient whom I have in mind displays a pleasing diffidence. But discharge makes for complications for such a patient if he expects to bed down with the Churchills and board with the Lyonses. Even a patient who is not deluded, but whose socialization and output of work is maintained only by constant pressure, is liable to be less well off if he leaves hospital for surroundings where comparable social pressures are not applied. In the past it was found that the long-stay patient who was discharged tended on the whole to do rather well – often better than the patient discharged after a short illness. The reason for this was that return to a family setting provided, at one time, an uplift so striking as to add to the patient's stability, whereas at the present stage of hospital improvement this alteration is not

so striking and indeed, if the family is too permissive and protective, the patient may deteriorate as a result of the move.
Enthusiastic discharging, then, provides a panacea for statisticians rather than patients.

On the credit side of this policy was the fillip given to occupational therapy. Most patients will work with their hands when
they go out. Old skills may be forgotten or obsolete, or the patient
may have become ill too early to have developed any expertise.
With the prospect of discharging many long-term patients
ahead, the therapeutic work given to patients started to become
more realistic in the sense of being more closely aligned with
the commonplace tasks of industry and the household. In a
typical hospital of the present day much of the occupational
therapy is concerned with increasing the confidence and skill
of long-rusticated housewives or reviving the manipulative
capacity of one-time workers. A premium is placed more on the
economic potentiality of the patient than on the pleasurable
nature of the task, not because the hospital exploits the patients
but in the hope that a proportion of the patients may become
capable of doing factory work. As much as possible these
patients operate in teams, so that incidental contact is provided
with their fellows, but the social aspect is, if anything, less
stressed than it was in the occupational therapy departments
of a decade ago.

This type of activity means that the occupational therapists
find themselves working with the most dilapidated patients and
their prestige is accordingly increased; if they succeed in training a patient to the point where he may be expected to undertake
industrial work, they pass him on to another therapeutic
organization within the hospital, usually run by nurses, where
products are manufactured on a contract basis for outside firms
in the course of *industrial therapy*. Here patients do real work,
and earn according to their output. Patients, especially smokers,
are chronically short of money in hospital in spite of their
official cash allowances, and the incentive to work at a competi-
tive rate is considerable. By the time the patient works his way
up to this level of occupation he is doing very different work
from that he enjoyed in the original kind of occupational

therapy department. Team tasks, with each member depending on the others for the maintenance of satisfactory output, are encouraged, but there is a temptation for the Industrial Therapy Officer, in his enthusiasm as a capitalist *manqué*, to pick the most profitable rather than the most intrinsically interesting and sociable of the contracts offered by interested firms: the patients' theoretical earnings on some tasks may exceed those of the nurse acting as Industrial Therapy Officer (a fact quoted with rueful pride by the nurse concerned).

The next stage in rehabilitation for those patients who speed up sufficiently, slowness being the main fault of chronic schizophrenic operatives, is working out of the hospital while sleeping within its walls. Many of the mental hospitals were built in open country, but few now have no factories close by. In times of full employment (upon which the success of this type of scheme is founded) jobs may usually be found. From there to discharge is a small enough step, if social conditions in the home are good. In cities dominated by a few large factories, the factories may themselves install machines for the benefit of such employees as are admitted.

The policy of discharging patients if this could be done, with a less cautious attitude to the possibility or probability of readmission, is not so urgently desirable, now that the hospitals are less fearsome, as it might have been a few years ago. This policy has contributed to the national statistics of the total population of mental hospitals which, it will be remembered, have been falling overall since 1955, here and abroad. In the discussion of the future of psychiatric services, undertaken later in the book (Chapter 6), it should be remembered that these figures reflect at once more and less than the therapeutic advances that seem to be their most obvious explanation.

THE COMMUNITY-BASED MENTAL HEALTH SERVICE

With more money, more psychiatrists, and governmental support the psychiatric services have been able to expand beyond the point at which, principally, they treated or tided over those patients who fell acutely ill and cared for the unfortunates who never recovered. At first the provision of any extra facility simply allowed a group of ill people who previously had not had any possibility of treatment to be seen and helped. When the voluntary status was statutorily instated in 1930 it led to a gradually increasing proportion of non-certified patients in hospitals, but the absolute number of certified patients entering annually stayed about the same; even allowing for population increase, the new voluntary patients were mostly drawn from a hitherto untreatable group. To a large extent the introduction of new facilities such as day-hospitals still means that patients who once could not undertake treatment can now do so, but the effect of the increased scope of the services has also been to improve the management of all patients seen.

All the forbidding aspects of the old mental hospitals helped the development of out-patient clinics. Memories of these aspects contributed to the enthusiasm with which vigorous discharge policies were adopted. Evidently, patients could not be discharged successfully in any numbers or with dispatch unless out-patient support were available. Patients discharged while taking maintenance doses of anti-schizophrenic or antidepressive drugs could not be left to take their pills regularly themselves (because, in general, patients do not) and needed surveillance if only for the purpose of adjustment of dosage levels. Chronic patients discharged to jobs among self-sufficient normal workmen needed support, advice, and early readmission if they showed signs of cracking under the multiple strains. The families of discharged patients needed advice and it was helpful, sometimes essential, for an ex-patient's home to be visited by a psychiatrist or social worker.

Out-patient facilities, centred on the hospital, came to offer much more than diagnosis and psychotherapy of the traditional kind. Some services were concentrated in what are called *day-hospitals*, where patients attend daily to receive treatment or, in some cases, company; these units vary widely in the patients they accommodate, some taking patients with psychoneuroses or personality problems, others mostly depressives or mostly old patients. From a tentative start in Russia before the war and

Montreal and London after the war, these units have spread until at present they are a feature of most psychiatric services, or are included in immediate plans. They are cheaper, in towns (where travelling is not a great part of the expense), than the provision of full hospital bed-facilities, and can do much the same in the way of therapy: they offer treatment to the patient whose family ties preclude admission but who is not suitable for occasional out-patient treatment. With the trend against cutting the patient off from community and normal work, complementary *night-hospitals* have sprung up, sometimes in the same premises: these units cater for patients who need some treatment or supervision of therapeutic activity, but who cannot or should not give up work to receive it.

Psychiatric *after-care* or *half-way hostels* are being set up to take care of the discharged patient who seems well enough in hospital but about whose chances of success outside some doubts are felt; these sound a more useful facility than they are: in practice, the patient who will do well does well without the need for a hostel and indeed is well advised to seek whatever accommodation is normal for him, while the patient whose future is in doubt may do better with his family. Nevertheless, for a few, including patients who positively depend on medication to keep them going and do not take it if left to themselves, patients without families and in need of ready-made social groups, patients who relapse suddenly without realizing it, and some others, these hostels are very suitable. Their establishment in a residential area constitutes an acid test of public enlightenment and is not always easy to bring about in the face of organized opposition from local ratepayers.

In the United States, as in certain localities in Scotland, Belgium, and elsewhere, *family care*, involving the enlistment of households willing to accommodate discharged patients while they find their feet, has been tried with some success; but partially recovered schizophrenics are more easily pitied in the imagination than in the flesh and it takes an exceptional family group to continue support for a patient to whom they have no ties of kin when little in the way of warmth or contact is included in the reward.

All these measures mean that the psychiatric patient in a progressive area receives good overall care whether he is in hospital or out. In some parts of the country the greater proportion of treatment is undertaken outside hospital, the patient continuing to reside at home and only being admitted for compelling social or medical reasons. By practising this policy vigorously at Worthing (the Worthing Experiment) Joshua Carse was able to reduce his admissions by 59 per cent, taking the load off a crowded mental hospital and at the same time giving better service to the patients seen. Other hospital-centred area organizations have not pursued his policy so whole-heartedly, but Carse's work has been influential and home-centred psychiatry is on the increase.

These medical and social changes, catalysed by the increased money available from government sources, have been abetted by the enlightened Mental Health Act of 1959, which encourages informality of admission and discharge and enjoins local authorities to cooperate in catering for the discharged and partially disabled psychiatric patient. These changes have also led to the framework of a system of care that is based on the community: the patient falls ill in the community and if possible he is treated there; if he leaves it, he does so only briefly and goes to a hospital organized so that it resembles in its informality and occupations the milieu from which he came. The United Kingdom is acting as a pathfinder in this administrative aspect of mental health, and the community-based mental health service is being instituted gradually in many areas of the United States, together with an open-door policy that is also based on the British plan, though opening the doors is proceeding more slowly than the provision of community-support facilities despite the cheapness of the former and the enormous expense of the latter.

All this sounds very hopeful, but nowhere in this country does more than the framework, with a few bits filled in, exist. In its entirety, the organization might prove impossibly expensive. The advantages of many parts of the system over the old one of admitting patients to hospitals are still under active debate. If past history is anything to go by, the present spate of public interest, the country's full employment and prosperity, the Government's provision of financial allocations for large-scale capital investment, and the great optimism of influential psychiatrists will not last. It is urgently necessary to decide which of the many measures pay off and which do not: which give a good return for money and time invested and which are unproductive. The humane reforms, whether or not they are any good as far as the pathology is concerned, psychiatrists gladly accept; about the others a great debate is going on. All the changes took place so rapidly, in orders so different in different hospitals, that no one can sort out with any precision what change had which effect.

6 The Future of Psychiatric Services

The reader may be willing to agree that the changes described in the last chapter are both radical and far-reaching but find, at the same time, that they are of less interest to him than the aspects of psychiatry that deal with quirks of personality, drinking patterns, or other topics with which he is more familiar. The author, too, prefers to consider the vagaries of individuals rather than kinks in graphs.

In the last ten years, however, it has been in the mental hospitals, not the academic units or the private clinics, that the great advances have taken place. The teaching hospitals are belatedly recognizing that this is so, and the more enterprising are trying to arrange liaison with mental hospitals in order that they may train their students and medical staff in modern therapeutic methods. If psychiatric practice in Britain is admired abroad it is for its contribution to mental hospital and community-care régimes, while for the patients of the future – readers and their children – the manner in which the methods and facilities evolve is of crucial importance. With this necessary explanation out of the way, it remains to consider what this future may hold.

One clear-cut statement of expectations does exist, and might well be used to bring order to what can only be an inconclusive discussion. This is the Hospital Plan,[1] put out by the Ministry of Health in early 1962, in which the future of all the hospitals in the country is decided on the basis of a detailed study of requirements and present facilities. A country that built no hospitals for a generation should be building hospitals, not

1. *A Hospital Plan for England and Wales*, Cmnd 1604, H.M.S.O., 1962.

making plans, but plans are cheaper and this one is most interesting.

Various statistical studies purport to show that the need for psychiatric beds will fall sharply over the next fifteen years. Because thirty years ago the schizophrenic stood only a 40 per cent chance of ever leaving hospital at all, while 87 per cent of these patients are now discharged within a year, because the influence of extended out-patient services, rehabilitation measures, early treatment and the other, mainly social, advances may be expected to increase their effect as they spread to all areas, and because the increased readmission rates (approximately quadrupled) are regarded merely as an aspect of the extension of community care, calculations can be made that show that the present chronic schizophrenic population is not being replaced, and that therefore the requirements of long-stay beds will fall to about 50 per cent (to take a typical estimate) of the present numbers.

The Minister's plan accepts that some such reduction is going to take place, and allows for a 50 per cent reduction in available beds over fifteen years. It follows that certain mental hospitals have been designated as destined to close, others have been earmarked for different uses (or have already, from 1962 on, been put to new uses), and still others are expected to reduce their numbers gradually over the fifteen-year period in question.

In place of the acute and chronic beds removed from the available pool by closure, the Minister proposes to provide psychiatric units at general hospitals, where thirty, sixty, or more beds will serve the local population for illnesses of short and medium length, the more chronic patients going to the mental hospitals that are still standing. These plans were made in the context of the Mental Health Act (1959), which allows the administrative equivalence of psychiatric and non-psychiatric hospital beds, and encourages (though it does not finance, as the most seriously intended Acts do) the local provision of community care. The Minister is therefore committed to the community-based psychiatric service, the idea of the dying mental hospital, the incorporation of psychiatry into the general hospital framework and belief in the reality of the basis of the figures that show reduction in chronicity. There is no reason to suppose that the plan is a rigid one, in the sense that the time-table is fixed, but the general tendencies are explicitly stated.

This plan understandably produced some startled reactions. Medical superintendents found, reading the paper one morning, that their hospitals were going to come down in a few years' time. Psychiatric hospital consultants, working harder than they ever had before, read incredulously of their decreasing patient-load. Some of the criticism came from the heart rather than the head, but most of it was factual.

To put it baldly, some psychiatrists do not believe that anything makes much difference to schizophrenia. An extreme exponent of this view would ascribe the whole of the reduction in the number of schizophrenics in hospital to temporary trends in management, admitting no increase in the rate of true remissions; he may quote articles such as one by F. S. Klaf and J. G. Hamilton, in which the clinical pictures and outcome of schizophrenics at the Bethlem hospital a century ago were compared with those seen today, and the proportion cured was found to be exactly the same. The writer dissociates himself from the strict view that schizophrenics are born, not made, and cannot be unmade, but accepts that much of the evidence on which a continuation of the fall in in-patient numbers is predicted is doubtful in the extreme.

Acutely schizophrenic patients are now more likely than not to be discharged within the year. They are also very likely to return (about 40 per cent) and rather more likely still to deteriorate, not necessarily to the point where readmission is needed (60 per cent). The chronically ill schizophrenics who have been rehabilitated and pharmacologically treated to the point where they are discharged do not necessarily do well outside hospital (if they all did well it would mean that the discharge policy was too conservative) but though less than 50 per cent may become self-supporting, 100 per cent of them are, of course, recorded as discharged, so that the latter raw figure, taken grossly, inflates the success.

The downward trend in national figures for occupied psychiatric beds still continues. But it may be that for any individual hospital there are only so many patients (acute and chronic) who can be discharged. A period of some years during which these were brought to the point at which discharge was practicable and humane would be a period during which, other things being equal, the figures for that hospital would fall; at the end of that time the fall would stop and might, if the discharged patients rebounded back into the hospital, reverse, to become the familiar upward progression of the hundred years that preceded 1955. An argument frequently heard is that this is precisely what is happening: the most progressive hospitals, who started the trend, have now reached the stage of stationary or rising figures, but, the bulk of the hospitals being still in the early phase of vigorous treatment and discharge, the total figures of the country as a whole still show a downward slope.

The discharge policy, however it may end, has had one good effect, that of reducing the overcrowding (7 per cent as late as 1959) in the mental hospitals, though schemes envisaged for modernizing the mental hospitals will lead automatically to an increase of 10 per cent on present overcrowding as wards are vacated for 'up-grading', even if the work is undertaken in a gradual fashion and spread over some years.

But the impact of the vigorous discharge policy on families and public has not yet been assessed. Word of mouth reports and a few studies have it that often discharge represents a hardship for the whole group involved: the patient may not only deteriorate but be aware of this and of his failure; the family are distressed by his oddities, behaviour disorders, and the social consequences of having the chronic patient present at entertainments, and in about a quarter of such families the distress is described as considerable. It is said that what is happening is that the acutely schizophrenic patient, tranquillized to the point of behavioural steadiness, trained to military standards of smartness, cleanliness, and punctuality, and group-pressured into leaving his symptoms out of conversations, shuttles backwards and forwards from hospital to family until, after the second or third experience of watching their own relative dilapidate despite all their efforts, the family refuses to have him return and the patient becomes chronic in the end, as ten years ago he would have been chronic from the beginning. The jibe that the open door has become the revolving door has some clinical judgement and administrative experience behind it, and if the implication is true it will turn out that it is not that the schizophrenic becomes chronic less often, but that he takes longer before he is declared so, producing confusion among the statistics and no benefit, now that chronic patients are treated so thoroughly, for the patient.

If the most optimistic discharge figures were true, in the sense of being reliable indications of what is really happening to the patients' disabilities, all that would be required for the Ministerial plan to work would be the organization needed to take care of the diverted load by other means, together with public goodwill. Public approval of the new liberal measures seems assured – at least that of the segment of the public whose voice is most often heard, and whose members incidentally contribute least to the pool of patients in need of good administration. But if all or most that the new discharge policies accomplish is the redistribution of the load of care and responsibility from the hospital to the family and local community, nothing above a book-keeping gain has been made, and the patience of the non-psychotic citizens will soon be exhausted. Lessons of the past show that the public reacts more violently to the misbehaviour of the insane than to the requests for tolerance that emanate from the mouths of reformers, and we must suppose that if the families and communities are pushed too far support will be withdrawn and this wave of professional enthusiasm will, like the others before it, break on the rocky shores of a legislature sensitive to public wishes.

The organization to be provided by the state will include out-patient facilities of unheard-of comprehensiveness, and the new general-hospital psychiatric beds. It is not certain that the out-patient departments, even if many psychiatrists are freed by the predicted (but not really predictable, after so short a statistical run) in-patient reductions, could ever be adequate to look after all the discharged patients, and certainly they can hardly undergo the required revolution in ten or twenty years. It is not that there are a whole lot of psychiatrists and social workers hanging around looking for something to do. Such psychiatrists as there are have their work cut out already and the psychiatric social workers are often more interested in and oriented by their training towards family and social problems of a psychoneurotic nature rather than the domiciliary management of emotionally unrewarding psychotic patients.

There is no sign that a great training programme is under way, or even planned: in fact, the staff situation looks like getting worse. Doctors may be going in for psychiatry to a lesser rather than a greater extent (this is certainly so in the United States). Adult psychiatric social work may lose some of its appeal as other lines in which a similar training may be used (probation work, work with children and so on) compete more openly for the few graduates that present or planned university places will produce. At the moment London offers some good psychiatric treatment, taking the average throughout the United Kingdom as a standard. But even here the supervision of the ex-patient is so poor that less than half take adequate dosages of drugs; only a very few are seen by a social worker; of the psychiatric out-patient clinics, 93 per cent are held in working hours.

When psychiatric staffing and the complement of social workers is inadequate the load can only be passed to the general practitioner, like so many of the other loads in medicine as a whole. The family doctor cannot be expected to detect early signs of relapse in the way that a psychiatrist of equal ability but greater experience can, and patients may slip excessively far before treatment is ordered or dosage adjusted. It is found that general practitioners, often economically minded whether the patient be private or State-aided, are more diffident than the psychiatrist when it comes to prescribing the rather massive-sounding dosages of drugs that psychiatric patients truly need, and so tend to prescribe inadequately and may even, if they read their drug-firm literature too trustingly, prescribe the wrong drugs. Psychiatrists cannot solve their problem of patient-load by passing it on to a body of men who already have 30 per cent of their patients presenting with emotional or other psychological difficulties and who, even without this segment of practice, have a greater case-load to bear.

T—F

Nevertheless, there is a lot to be said for incorporating the general practitioner fully into the community-based scheme. He is one of the pillars of the community concerned. He may know a great deal about the individual family situation to which the patient reacts, though, with a list of three or four thousand patients, this often-quoted advantage is usually less substantial than it appears to the hospital consultant. He is one of the very few official or authority figures that may command the respect of the lower (working, labouring, social class V) classes who contribute so many schizophrenic subjects to the national total. But if he is to play a full part he must receive a more comprehensive training in psychiatry at the medical schools. There are signs that one day he will, but the recent cutbacks on university grants, among other things, have put this day off by a long while (see also Chapter 5).

All that is left to mention is the proposal that general hospitals should provide many of the beds for psychiatric in-patients, for which there is much to be said. Emotionally, psychiatrists will gain from incorporation into a general hospital organization. The psychiatrist may have chosen his line because it takes him as far as possible from laboratories, pus, and blood, but he is more likely to have undertaken the speciality for the particular closeness and responsibility it allows and enjoins.

The psychiatrist is often aware that he is no match as an organic diagnostician for the physicians and neurologists with whom he comes into professional contact, but at the same time he likes to keep his weapons bright by polishing them in good company and may feel, as a man who can diagnose some organic conditions by signs more subtle (and therefore earlier) than those commonly used by neurologists, that he has something in the way of skill to teach his colleagues. Also, he is anxious to be useful: there are many occasions when calling in a psychiatrist will make sense of a nonsensical case or allow the treatment to be improved out of all recognition. This is not to say that psychiatrists expect or would wish to be called in for every psychological or social problem that comes up in a general medical ward, for general physicians are as competent to deal with stress-reactions and domestic complications as their opposite numbers in psychiatry. Nor, in a teaching hospital, does it mean that the psychiatrist would wish to take over instruction in the management of doctor–patient relationships or the patients' reactions to the threats of illness and cure, except by default, for here again the doctor actually managing the patients is the best instructor on them and, if he is willing to talk on psychological subjects, will teach more effectively than a psychiatrist visiting the wards only occasionally and possessing no clinical responsibility for the patients in question.

Reintegration into general hospital work would mean a real promotion for psychiatry. There is no doubt that it is a branch of medicine that commands less respect within the profession than without. It is not certain why this should be so: but it is, after all, easy to succeed in psychiatry, and some who do well would have done less well in a line where results could be more precisely measured; some strange people go in for it; and the patients whom psychiatrists see are seldom in danger of death in the direct way that surgical patients may be. Nevertheless, there are important reasons why even modest psychiatrists wish that the speciality was treated less like a totally destitute relation (about 14 per cent of consultant psychiatrists received monetary merit awards in 1951, compared with 67 per cent of neurologists).

For those already in psychiatry, this does not matter vitally to themselves. What does matter is that the opinions doctors in general hold about a speciality decide to a large extent the quality of the postgraduate recruits; and psychiatry, whatever it may once have been, now provides some of the most vigorous therapeutic programmes and easily the most baffling and therefore, presumably, the most subtle, of the biochemical-genetic problems of the age. It follows that high intellectual quality is needed in the younger psychiatrists, who will only be attracted in the first place if the speciality is approved by the rest of the profession. If the psychiatrists of the present day are not to be cut off from general hospitals of the future as they were in the past, their standards and therefore their standing will inevitably rise.

At first sight, then, the suggestion that the more acute psychiatric beds should be housed in general hospitals is a welcome one. But there are many practical difficulties. Psychiatric patients have different requirements from those in general wards: the reduction in administrative distinctions between psychiatric and non-psychiatric patients does not mean that they are really alike. The once popular idea that most psychiatric patients could be treated in a general ward, mixed with medical patients, is so much nonsense. If psychiatric units are to be set up within their walls, the organization of the general hospitals concerned is going to alter radically. For one thing, psychiatric patients are mostly up and about. If they are to be treated as well as they would be in a mental hospital (and one hopes that at least that standard will be reached) they need facilities for occupation and the relief of boredom. Therefore, in terms of space, especially valuable urban ground-space, these patients will have to receive more than their nominal due of what the site and building can offer. Psychiatric patients should not be expected to keep to the rather military rules that general hospitals impose on the patients who, by entering their walls, join a continuous tradition that had its origins in poor-law or charity; so the rules must be relaxed.

Some psychiatric patients – 2 or 3 per cent – will need custodial care for a few days after admission, but most will not, and when there is some doubt the psychiatrist may decide that it will be in the patient's interests that a justifiable risk should be taken. It follows that, in the matter-of-fact phrase of a recent leading article, 'an occasional suicide must be expected'. To the established medical and nursing interests of a general hospital the psychiatric patients, looking robustly healthy, spending much of their time loafing about, taking their own discharges if they feel like it and being readmitted if they change their minds, often complaining or indifferent and occasionally killing themselves, are likely to compare unfavourably with the brave and disciplined ranks of patients offering themselves for surgery, and may therefore be unwelcome guests. Some of the staff's emotional problems, of very high voltage and great duration, noted in psychiatric hospitals when some of the wards were free and easy (along the ward-community lines described earlier) while some remained hierarchical, are likely to be repeated in general hospitals harbouring new psychiatric units of any size.

Yet, if psychiatric treatment is to be done properly, the psychiatric wards must be different and, as it would seem, privileged: in the planning of these hospitals, if they come about, it is to be hoped that the psychiatrists, despite their low prestige, will be able to insist on their own specifications.

In-patient units have been tried on a small scale already, notably in teaching hospitals. The results produced by these units compared very favourably with those produced by the mental hospitals. Since they took (and take) patients of good prognosis, treat them intensively and as far as medical time is concerned prodigally, and draw their clients mainly from the middle and upper classes (a reflection of the anxiety of general practitioners that their more sensitive patients should not go to mental hospitals) – these classes carrying better prognoses for reasons incompletely elucidated – their results, though certainly good, are not truly comparable. The point has been made that if they received patients whose principal need was resocialization and training they would need to reorganize so as to resemble more closely the modern mental hospital if their results were to continue to bring them credit. If the general hospital units increased and expanded to take over the acute work of the mental hospitals a new factor, that of competition for staff, would enter into the situation. There has always been some competition to work for a time at the teaching hospital in-patient units, partly because of the training provided but also because of the prestige of the great hospitals and the pleasant conditions of work. If more than half the work, and that half the more immediately interesting, is transferred to general hospitals the staffing of the remote and by then entirely chronic units will probably become even more unsatisfactory than it is today.

The changes in psychiatric services over the last generation have been reviewed and the plans based on these have been described and critically examined. It has been easy, as always, to be sourly destructive; perhaps, in reality, the governmental plans will be put into practice and not shelved again because of financial stringency; perhaps community-care really is more like a panacea than a humanitarian surge that may go too far;

perhaps general hospital units will provide advantages for patients as well as psychiatrists. But we do not, and cannot, know.

The last statement is not empty nihilism: it contains the roots of action. Not only do we not know about the effectiveness of the measures we have recently undertaken, but we do not know what therapies we shall have in the future. Psychiatry is not like the study of infectious disease. We cannot say fairly confidently, as bacteriologists once could, that treatment being available for half the illnesses concerned, treatment (including prevention) for the rest would come about after a suitable investment of time and trouble along lines already laid down and practically proved. In psychiatry we think our measures probably work: we reckon to treat a good half of the patients fairly well; we do not know why the treatments produce their capricious effects. Practically all of them were chance discoveries, and no promising lines of proven utility in psychiatry are being followed up that may be expected to revolutionize morbidity.

It is the complete ignorance of the future that points the way to the type of planning that is needed. Obviously, in a speciality with three or four illnesses making up the overwhelming majority of the clinical material seen, a cure for one of these or a gross increase in another would upset the whole of the planning unless the keynote of it all were *flexibility*.

It is right that psychiatric patients should be treated with the same organizational whole as general medical and surgical patients. It is not right that patients who become chronic should be excluded from this type of hospital, which would quickly become the *élite* segment of hospital services. It is appropriate for some psychiatric patients to have laboratory and radiological facilities of the greatest modernity and scope near at hand, though most of them will not need extensive investigation at an instrumental level. Advances may alter the proportions needing and not needing complicated investigations; it is worth remembering that most recent advances have led to greater rather than lesser complexity of investigational and therapeutic methods, and comparable advances in psychiatry, where most of the simple ideas have already been tried, will presumably follow the same pattern. How can these unknown and impermanent requisites be flexibly provided for?

In an article that seems to me the most far-sighted statement of the many that have appeared in medical journals on the topic of hospital planning, T. McKeown suggests that patients should be classified not according to their illnesses, but their personal and individual therapeutic needs. According to the figures of his survey, only 54 per cent of all patients need full facilities – meaning heavy nursing, piped oxygen and suction, non-stop operating theatres, doctors permanently available at a few seconds' notice, and so on. Some of the patients, but not many, in wards with full facilities would be primarily psychiatric, and would include the delirious, the suicidal, the acutely or dangerously ill, and possibly, if new treatments call for it, those under some intensive or hazardous therapy. About 9 per cent of the patients of all diagnostic types need 'limited physical facilities'. Again, a few of these patients would be primarily psychiatric – patients with physical disabilities or complicating organic illnesses for whom some routine care is needed – though most would be sufferers from arthritic conditions and the like.

Thirty-one per cent of all the patients in an area need 'limited mental facilities' of whom most would, of course, be primarily long-term psychiatric patients, though some might be patients with rehabilitation problems after long disablement from trauma or disease. Six per cent, the remainder, are in hospital for social reasons. Whether these last patients are called psychiatric or not is all according to taste: they are admitted under the care of whoever saw that it was necessary, and the speciality of the consultant in charge is less relevant than his perspicacity.

McKeown proposes the provision of a *balanced hospital community*, with about half the buildings suitable for acute patients with all that modern treatments and diagnostic methods entail in the way of auxiliary personnel and equipment. The rest of the buildings, grouped around the acute core, would resemble residential accommodation rather than the typical hospital wards of today and would, therefore, be vastly less expensive. In these wards, providing limited facilities, internal structural permanence could be kept to a minimum, allowing for changes of use if treatment advances rendered the provision of any particular kind of care obsolete. If all these buildings were on one site (and if hostels or social advances in the country took care of the 6 per cent at present taking up hospital beds because of social difficulties), if nurses and medical staff either rotated or had patients both in the acute (full facilities) and sub-acute or chronic (limited facilities) parts, then the problems of prestige, differential interest, training, staffing, and the isolation of chronic patients would be removed: the expense of providing separate laboratories and radiological departments for psychiatric hospitals, and conversely of providing 'acute' standards of care for those chronically physically ill would be sharply reduced.

I would suggest that McKeown's scheme is the one most likely to save us from posterity's strictures: it is rational and based on easily confirmed facts. It promises, at only a slightly increased capital cost, a comprehensive system of in-patient care for all the sick of a neighbourhood, without differentiating against those unfortunate enough to have certain types of illness or unhappily failing to respond to treatment. In the United Kingdom, with all health services centrally controlled by one Minister and the climate of public and professional opinion ideal for reform, we have a unique opportunity to set the style for a century to come. Over-reliance on the modish medical régimes of the day will make a poor foundation for so important a structure as the hospital services of the land.

Pavlov: The Revival
7 of Interest

The failure of Freudian methods to live up to the exaggerated expectations of the stricter disciples led to much casting about for alternative schools of thought among those who find it helpful to belong to one, while experimental psychologists found little in Freudian psychology that could be incorporated into their hard-won knowledge or tested by the methods they used. They continued their painstaking attempts to establish laws of behaviour for animals and men. The behaviourist psychologists studied processes of learning extensively, and many of the statements they made about the manner in which a subject's responses were altered by past experience corresponded closely to the laws established by Pavlov, whose views had already been subjected to some clinical trial of an uncritical but large-scale kind, because of the incorporation of Pavlovian dogma into the dialectic materialist foundations of Soviet psychiatry.

Pavlov was the winner of a Nobel Prize long before he started to study the functions of the central nervous system. His work on digestion, his original physiological interest, gradually became more subtle, and at last he began to find that the psychological states and past experiences of his experimental animals were rendering his experiments useless, in so far as they were aimed at elucidating facts about glands in the alimentary tract. He could not tell, for instance, which of two powders placed on the tongue caused a greater flow of saliva if the animal's flow started at the sight of the experimenter and varied in volume and constituents according to how the animal felt about the situation in general and that day's work in particular.

Other experimenters had met similar snags but had taken

refuge in vague generalities about the animal's mental state and accepted the inaccuracies. Pavlov, on the other hand, recognized that his work had reached the barrier of the brain and determined to bring some scientific order to this sphere of physiological activity. The story of his work, with the elaborate techniques used, the hardships undergone by his team during the food shortages, the special status granted to Pavlov by the revolutionary government, and the brilliant results that were the final reward, need not be told again.

Pavlov tried to keep his work strictly factual and non-speculative, but the urgent needs of psychiatric patients made him feel bound to try to fit his results into the knowledge that existed about psychoses. As a result, he made some diffident theorizations about psychopathology that were taken too seriously by his followers and were undoubtedly premature.

The fact that his work is sometimes over-valued cannot disguise the quality of his principal discoveries. His work was intended to produce an account of the reflexes of the brain corresponding in its accuracy to that available for the spinal cord, and he started with an examination of the built-in reflexes, particularly those concerned with salivation (which allowed of quantitative measurements). These inborn reflexes he called unconditioned, to distinguish them from reflexes acquired later. He then showed that if the unconditioned stimulus (such as an object placed in the mouth) was accompanied by some neutral stimulus such as the sound of a bell on each occasion that it was presented to the experimental animal, the bell came to have a significance for the animal corresponding approximately to that of the unconditioned stimulus. Thenceforth the bell, the conditioned stimulus, would precipitate a reflex flow of saliva even in the absence of the original unconditioned stimulus.

His work, once the original formulation was made, was directed towards determining the laws governing these conditioned reflexes, their mode of formation and extinction, and their characteristics.

Obviously, the conception provided a way in which an organism's response to the environment and moulding by circumstances could be comprehended in an orderly way. Pavlov called the simple sensory stimuli, such as the bells, the 'first signalling system', these stimuli indicating to the animal that this or that unconditioned stimulus was imminent. He pointed out that man's use of symbols such as words provided him with a 'second signalling system', enabling reflexes to be modified by the incorporation of ideas and concepts as well as the classical conditioning undergone by the rest of the animal kingdom. This elaboration allowed further insights: neuroses and behaviour disorders may be regarded as sets of faulty conditioned reflexes, and psychotherapy as modifications of the complex of reflexes by use of the second signalling system.

These ideas were particularly influential in Russia, where Freud's premises are regarded as too arbitrary and the roots of neurosis are thought to be found in current social circumstances rather than the events of early childhood; if manifest symptoms rather than predisposition are principally investigated, this is almost certainly true, and the Soviet concentration on current stresses in the treatment of minor mental illness has probably been both economic and effective. Pavlov's speculations about the role of conditioned reflex psychology, including its aberrations, in the functional psychoses have not led to equivalent therapeutic benefit, most probably because they are oversimplifications, but there are occasional reports that schizophrenic-like states have been produced in the course of intensive brain-washing (another technique which, though partly Russian traditional-empirical, has been tidied up by the application of Pavlovian techniques) and the theories, though untenable in their present form, cannot be entirely discarded.

Investigation by Hull and others into the processes of learning, a topic of great theoretical interest and practical importance, went on during the same period. Learning may be said to take place when an organism modifies its behaviour as a consequence of events in its life; and clearly such a definition would include the development of conditioned reflexes, so that experimental work on learning might be expected to show some overlap with Pavlov's studies.

It seems that learning of a precision type does not usually

take place by means of classical Pavlovian conditioning, but by means of a complementary mechanism known as 'operant' or 'instrumental' conditioning. The animal developing a Pavlovian conditioned response to a bell does so in a passive manner: the bell achieves significance because it is closely associated in time with the unconditioned stimulus provided by the food placed in the animal's mouth. The animal developing an operant conditioned reflex, on the other hand, participates in the process: for example, a rat moved by drives and appetites makes various random and exploratory movements if placed in a cage, and if one of the movements, such as that which depresses a small pedal, is constantly followed by the appearance of a pellet of food, the animal learns to press the pedal when it is hungry. The process is one of trial and error, initiated by the animal's drives and completed because the significant activity, that of pressing the pedal, results in a *reduction in drive* – in this case, that of hunger.

The incorporation of the idea of drive into the scheme of learning and conditioning was not only useful in advancing the theory but in accordance with general experience. It allowed some speculations, rather more precise than usual, to be made about the role of learning in the production of neurosis.

Neurotic symptoms, it was suggested, may be thought of as the consequence of faulty learning. Anxiety is the central neurotic symptom and may itself be an inappropriate response to stimuli, perhaps mislearnt early on by means of classical conditioning (which, when concerned with autonomic functions, shows remarkable durability). Alternatively or additionally, neurotic symptoms may be learnt (in the operant, or instrumental manner) because of their capacity to lower anxiety; that is, to reduce drive, anxiety operating as drive whether normal or neurotic. Anxiety-reducing neurotic symptoms are pathological because they do not deal with the source of the anxiety and are therefore inefficient, but they quickly become established because they produce a temporary reduction in anxiety on each occasion that they are used, a reduction that reinforces the conditioned reflex and perpetuates the neurotic behaviour.

Thus neurotic manifestations are not regarded as symptoms

of some deep-seated malaise, but as the illness itself. The anxiety was either the result of faulty learning or, if justifiable, cannot be dealt with rationally because neurotic methods (i.e. counting or hand-washing rituals) have become habitual. The implications for treatment are obvious: what has been learned must be unlearned or, put in the usual way, faulty conditioning must be annulled by deconditioning.

In a broad way, this is just restating the obvious. Most sophisticated psychotherapy has as its aim the extinction of old inappropriate and uncomfortable patterns of response and the substitution of new; and speech, the second signalling system, is exploited for its convenience and speed. There is no special use in thinking of psychotherapy in terms of learning theory, rather than in terms of what have become classical psychodynamics, because whatever his frame of reference, the psychotherapist does much the same in the consulting room. But certain syndromes lend themselves very readily to deconditioning techniques, and many of them respond poorly to other methods, including prolonged psychotherapy.

The best-known and most fully authenticated of the successful applications of learning and conditioned reflex theory has been in the treatment of bed-wetting. The child who wets the bed at night has failed to develop the conditioned response of wakefulness to a high tension in the bladder wall. Training methods do not seem to affect the incidence of nocturnal enuresis, and the frequent presence of a family history of late establishment of nocturnal continence indicates that the error is constitutional; it probably consists of a low capacity to condition. The rational treatment therefore consists of the provision of a series of learning experiences, encouraging the linkage, along classical lines, of high pressure in the bladder with both closure of the sphincters and waking up.

In parts of West Africa this is accomplished by placing a certain type of snail on the inside of the thigh, this snail staying immobile when dry but starting to move at once when wetted; the moving snail wakes the child and it is credibly reported that, as a conditioning stimulus, the sensation is hard to beat.

The equivalent of this method in paediatric work is the

'Mowrer' bell and pad apparatus. This consists of an open electric circuit incorporating an electric bell, which is closed when urine is passed; the bell rings and the child wakes. The method is convenient and effective and is widely quoted as being confirmatory for the theories of the learning school of therapists, especially since eradication of the symptom is not followed by the advent of further symptoms, as theories relating the bed-wetting to deeper causes would seem to require.

The method just described is not one of deconditioning, but of hastening the initial conditioning. It is applied to a group of children whose capacity to condition is low. Now if, as is probable, the capacity to condition is a personality characteristic showing the usual type of distribution, it would be reasonable to look for other examples of poor or slow conditioning, in the hope that similar treatment might be used. Conditioning is of great importance in the development of social conformity, and some correlations have been found between capacity to condition and conventionality. The subject who always does the right thing socially, never forgets a birthday, and punctiliously returns hospitality is likely, on the whole, to be a creature of habit and routine, and to condition easily. The person at the opposite pole, who conforms sporadically or not at all, probably conditions poorly and if his social inconsiderateness is extreme may be called psychopathic.

One way of regarding psychopaths, then, is as subjects who need more frequent and more emphatic learning experiences before conduct is modified: this gives coherence to many of the methods used in the management of this type of personality disorder and offers guidance, admittedly not of a very original kind, to those attempting to deal with habitual offenders against the law.

The failures to condition that have just been described cause inconvenience to those in the patient's circle. It is excessive or faulty conditioning that causes most discomfort for the patient. The most characteristic neurotic condition that qualifies for deconditioning therapy is the phobic state: a tense and obsessional person, beset by anxiety because of current personal difficulties and never entirely at ease in a crowd may find, when first surrounded by people after the recent increase in background anxiety, that the usual increase in tension brought about by being hemmed in causes her to notice, for the first time, symptoms of overt anxiety amounting to fear. If the nature of her duties calls for return to the crowded location, and she returns half a dozen times before the true cause of her increased level of anxiety is dealt with or disperses, she is likely to develop a conditioned response of anxiety-attacks to the stimulus provided by large groups of people. It is possible, if the first attack was severe, for conditioning to occur without repetition of the stimulus at all.

Once the patient develops an irrational and recurrent fear of non-threatening stimuli, she may be said to have a phobic state. From then on the patient is frequently too preoccupied with her phobic symptoms and the precautions she must take to prevent them to attend to her real problems; furthermore her conditioned anxiety is likely to extend by association so that not only crowds but places in which crowds congregate become threatening, and enclosed spaces, open spaces, and public means of transport are barred to her, the most extreme development of the phobic system leading to a house-bound state. Such a patient makes heroic attempts, spurred on both by her own awareness of the ridiculous nature of her fear and the hearty advice of those in her circle who have not suffered similar symptoms, to face the fear-producing situations and master the weakness; these attempts simply provide confirmatory learning experiences, since panic regularly supervenes. The patient is trapped.

The therapeutic aim is to get rid of the conditioned reflexes concerned in these symptoms. There are several means by which, theoretically, this may be brought about; the reflexes will ultimately diminish by disuse, so that the house-bound patient who capitulates would, perhaps after years, lose the phobias, but the most prompt and practical method of annulling the reflex is by instituting another, incompatible response to the stimuli: this is done by inducing in the patient a tendency to relax whenever faced by an object for which she has a phobia.

An illustration is necessary. The patient has a series of

phobic objects, some grossly frightening and others mildly anxiety-producing. The patient who fears crowds and open places may be able, with little difficulty, to hang her clothes out in the garden. It would be impossible to induce the patient to relax in the Albert Hall or a lift, but she might manage to do so in the garden, if suitably influenced. In the actual therapeutic situation the patient could be taught how to relax at will, then induced to do so while thinking of a short walk in the garden, then encouraged to take an actual walk, relaxing consciously while it continues. With gradual progress, a series of connexions are made, associating relaxation with phobic situations so that the two reflexes cancel out. The approach used is cautious and slow, but much more effective than methods used by the unaided patient.

Learning-theorists interested in therapy sometimes claim that treatment of this kind makes psychotherapy of the conventional variety unnecessary, and much polemic has scarred the polished scientific articles written on this subject. In reviewing the course of this type of treatment the resemblance to the usual type of verbal therapy cannot be denied, however, for much support and encouragement is given by the therapist; also, at the end of the course, the original anxiety, if it persists, must be examined and the reasons the patient had for burying it rather than dealing with its source considered and discussed.

Deconditioning therapy has been used in a variety of other psychiatric conditions. Fetishism, homosexuality, writer's cramp, tics and other abnormal states have been described as benefiting, while alcoholism is commonly treated by inducing aversion to a range of alcoholic beverages. The impact of learning theory on the treatment of these and other conditions has been beneficial, making for a greater concentration on precise techniques and critical examination of results.

The high hopes of the more ardent proponents of the method have not been completely fulfilled, in the event, even allowing for the usual fall in success-rates as a treatment loses its novelty; and though psychologists put some of the failures down to technical failures and departures from the requirements of conditioned-reflex theory, treatments must be judged by their results in practice; also the number of patients who can be treated principally by deconditioning techniques is rather small, for phobic and allied states are not common compared with other psychiatric conditions, and the results reported in homosexuality, alcoholism, and motor disorders are either patently unreliable or unconfirmed.

Research into learning theory has been stimulated by its possible applications in psychiatry, and it is now one of the most comprehensively mapped of the sub-sections of psychology, with applications in learning machines and other training devices appearing with great frequency. Psychiatry, though at present unable to exploit the theory to the full in the realm of psychoneurosis and behaviour disorder, has found many of the principles useful in other tasks, notably the retraining of the chronic populations of the country's mental hospitals. It is to be hoped that, however the idea may be resisted by the respective devotees, the learning-theory views on the psychopathology of the psychoneuroses and Freudian insights into the same dynamics may be blended into a consistent theory at some future date, a theory more scientific than Freud's and less starkly mechanistic than that evolved from Pavlov and Hull.

8 Personality Deviations

The difference between the psyche of the patient and that of the non-patient may be very large or very small. When it is very small the only clear-cut difference that may be discerned between the patient and the non-patient is that the patient elected to present himself to a doctor. It is with these patients, who closely resemble normal people, that this chapter is concerned.

A patient may attend a psychiatrist, or be persuaded by his friends to attend, and say that his trouble is that he has always been different from and in some ways worse than other people. If he means that he has some internal psychological characteristic or some aspect of habitual behaviour that is normal enough in its quality but abnormal in its quantity, such as that he has too much aggression or is pitifully lacking in this trait, he may well be describing what is called a personality deviation. For this to be the case the disorder must be fixed and permanent and if questioning establishes that this is so, the label of personality deviation may be attached:

A fifty-year-old man was referred to a psychiatrist on the initiative of his personnel officer, who felt that the man was so unusually timid that he must have something wrong with him. The patient was an only son, was brought up by his widowed mother in a grossly over-protective way, and never had friends of his own. He left the local school and went to a local office (Civil Service); he always lived in the same house, he always worked at the same job, and he never went away for a holiday. His hobby was going in for newspaper competitions but during the late nineteen-fifties he started looking at television on occasion and became quite interested in sports such as football, which he had not previously seen. His work record was excellent; he had refused promotion within his clerical grade lest he be required to take more responsibility, so that an apparent lack of advancement was self-imposed. He was too shy to say good morning to his colleagues, some of whom he had known for thirty years, and when he walked down the corridor he moved sideways lest his eyes met those of another. It was this last characteristic, taken in conjunction with his extreme nervousness in all situations, that caught the attention of the personnel officer. A 'diagnosis' of personality deviation (inadequate, anxiety prone) was made but no treatment was offered since the patient was evidently surprised that anyone should consider that he was ill, and had no wish to change; he recognized that he was different from some others he knew, and admitted that he might have missed out on certain aspects of life but pointed out with unwonted firmness that he had always been the same, and he was not complaining.

Evidently, since nobody corresponds to the ideal normal, every person in the world may be said to have a personality deviation of some degree, present company excepted. However, the standard of normality used is not that of the ideal normal, but the statistical normal. This means that every quality is taken to have a variable level in human beings, most subjects possessing a given quality in some near-average degree; only those who are so unusually heavily endowed with, or deprived of, the quality as to become misfits or miserable have personality problems of an overt kind; and of these only the proportion that offer themselves for therapy, whether willingly or not, become psychiatric charges, since psychiatrists do not seek them out.

To revert to the example of aggression, only patients so aggressive as constantly to be tormented by the desire to hack at their local minorities (Jews, Negroes, white people, etc.) or who get into endless brawls would be regarded as pathologically aggressive, though lesser degrees would be noticed in a psychiatrist's diagnosis. In the same way, only patients who were unable to say boo to a shackled goose, or to assert themselves to the mildest degree in propitious circumstances would be regarded as pathologically deficient in aggression, though here again lesser degrees would be noticed.

It will be seen that the scientific study of personality is concerned at the start with the description of normal personalities and the delimitation of abnormalities, and that the essential basis of this work is statistical. From this purely psychological aspect, personalities are abnormal if they are highly unusual, and the question of whether the particular abnormality is useful or harmful is, though interesting, irrelevant. A scientific classification would probably begin by distinguishing between normal and abnormal along mathematical lines. For the patient, on the other hand, the important question is whether his personality is suitable for the demands he, in his particular environment, makes on it. If it is not, then even if it could be regarded in the scientific sense as coming within the normal range, he will complain of difficulties associated with relative deficiencies in his personality and will be diagnosed as suffering from a personality problem. *offering unwanted advice*

The fifty-year-old patient previously described and noted on his first appearance as having a personality deviation consisting principally of inadequacy and anxiety-proneness, later came to the psychiatrist's attention again. Some years after his first visit, at which he and the psychiatrist had agreed that any attempt at treatment would be officious, the patient became blind. Under this extra stress the patient's deficiencies, to which he had previously been able to adapt by severely limiting his activities, became for the first time a problem for him: that is to say, his personality deviation now constituted a personality problem.

This is the practical psychiatrist's way of thinking of personality deviations, the importance of which, for him as for his patients, depends on the amount of discomfort they cause, regardless of their scientific status. The question of personality deviations having advantages seldom or never arises, since patients do not attend psychiatrists to say how well they are. Lastly, to complete the list of ways in which personality variations can affect those concerned, the point of view of the public must be considered. For those who wish to go about their business undisturbed, the only kinds of personality that prove socially disrupting are those that cause their owners to behave in a disorderly or otherwise anti-social way. For the general public the prototypical personality deviation must be that of the man who gives free rein to destructive and other anti-social impulses outside his home:

motive for help

A twenty-two-year-old patient was admitted for investigation of his mental state pending prosecution. He came from a well-to-do family and had been expensively educated at a suspiciously large number of well-known schools. Despite good physical condition and high intelligence he had spent much of his National Service in detention and the whole of it as a private soldier; by dint of employing his fellow-soldiers as proxies he had never done a single guard duty. After leaving the army he made no attempt to work, but instead undertook a series of delinquent activities. He regularly stole fast cars, driving them until the tanks were almost empty and sometimes returning them at this stage to the parking-places he took them from, with the intention, later fulfilled, of stealing them again when the owners had put more petrol in. He took up with undesirable associates and carried offensive weapons. He stole goods and sold them at pawn-brokers' shops. All his activities were done for his immediate benefit, on impulse and without planning, so that for a delinquent act to take place it was enough that a wish should occur to him. He was caught in the act of selling a tape-recorder that he had stolen, having failed to take precautions that a normal steady criminal with half his intelligence would have reckoned elementary. This patient was considered to be a psychopath.

There is remarkable lack of agreement about the meaning of the word *psychopath*, and even the usual connotation of disapproval is not entirely constant, as evinced by the well-known professional plate reading 'Osteopath, Homoeopath, Psychopath'. The three possible viewpoints about personality deviation give a clue about the cause of the ambiguity; for the word psychopath has been used to describe personality deviations of the scientific and the practical medical as well as the anti-social (sociopathic) variety, dissimilar though these are.

An attempt will be made in this chapter to sort out what has gradually become a vexed and confused topic, but the use of the term psychopath will be reserved throughout for those who (1) have a personality deviation and (2) undertake activity as a reflection of the deviation that is in some way socially disruptive and excites disapproval.

THE STUDY OF PERSONALITY

The scientific study of personality, as undertaken by psychologists, is of primary importance in our understanding of all personality problems, but it is not at present a sphere in which enough work has been done to provide a good grounding for our clinical work. In part, this is because much of the basic research must be done on subjects with normal personalities, and though many patients have perfectly normal personalities before their illnesses start, few of our patients display normal personality characteristics at the time they are seen. The clinical material for the research is lacking.

Much of the clinical work that has been done has been along the familiar lines of verbal description. There has also been a tendency to seek dichotomy, or a series of dichotomies, such as dominant/submissive, as if to satisfy a human need for black/white distinctions. Much of the clinical descriptive work done has been of very high quality and a knowledge of it, together with a working acquaintance with great literature, enables most psychiatrists to sum up patients' personalities in a few evocative phrases: unfortunately vividness of description does not necessarily make for scientific worth.

The various dichotomies, of which Jung's famous extraversion and introversion is the best known example, have widened our range of description rather than divided our patients sharply into classes, but some of them are proving to correspond to psychological test results, of which more will be said shortly. It is unlikely that further descriptive work will be done representing a great advance on what has been achieved already, and for further progress we must seek elsewhere; the results of this clinical research are respectable, even formidable, and some of the types described will also probably prove to have a scientific basis in objectively measurable traits and reaction-patterns when this part of the work is done.

It is now generally agreed that certain personality-types, meaning subjects in whom a constellation of traits produces a distinctive total picture, are more prone to certain psychiatric illnesses than the generality of the populace. The most widely accepted examples of this connexion are between the cyclothymic personality (meaning jovial and warm) and manic-depression, and the schizothymic personality (meaning, in brief, withdrawn and cool) and schizophrenia. Such personalities, in the clinical frame of reference, are noteworthy solely because of their association with overt illness but the fact that they can be distinguished means that, scientifically, they are deviations.

If present to a more marked degree, the characteristics of the schizothymic and cyclothymic personalities may produce discomfort or adaptational difficulties, when the personalities are commonly called schizoid or cycloid to distinguish them from the harmless variants they resemble. A whole series of abnormal personality types has been described by European writers, and though the medical interests of the authors make for a concentration on those subjects whose quirks cause trouble of one kind or another, the comprehensive classifications that are the fruits of this clinical research are probably the nearest we shall get to a satisfactory verbal description of personality groupings. In the best-known of the clinical classifications, Kurt Schneider lists the hyperthymic (happy-go-lucky), depressive, fanatic, attention-seeking (hysterical), labile (with rapid intense mood-changes), explosive (with short-circuit reactions of rage or despair under stress similar to those seen in pre-adult life), affectionless (without remorse or shame), weak-willed, and asthenic (permanently weak) personalities; together with the insecure personalities, who may be excessively sensitive, or obsessional and inclined to protective rituals.

Even this exhaustive survey, like many lesser ones, provides only a list. Few personalities seen in clinical work (or socially) fit one or other category very closely and to most of them several of the descriptions could apply in some degree. Clinically determined 'types' are probably most useful when their identification allows some induction to be made about the illness to which such a subject is liable, and the elaboration of many types and sub-types without such pathological connexions is an exercise that can continue indefinitely because of the infinite combinations of characteristics that make up the individualities of the human race.

Psychiatric preoccupation with description and classification may seem to be excessive, but it is not until some satisfactory and consistent system is worked out that research into causation and assessment of the results of treatment can be seriously or successfully attempted. The use of verbal descriptions makes for interesting case-histories but a study of clinical records with a view to finding what subtle factors in early life made what subtle differences in adult personality is almost bound to fail: one psychiatrist sees aggression everywhere, another finds only obsessionals, and such studies are often more useful in weighing the psychiatrists than their clinical material. The most important recent development in the study of personality has been connected with escape from the linguistic strait-jacket: there is no justification for supposing that descriptive words refer to real entities in the central nervous system or that, if they do, the entities are single ones.

Assessment of personality at interview is done by finding out, preferably from both the patient and at least one other, how the patient has reacted to various situations and stresses in his life, particularly those that are common or peculiarly testing. If a type is discerned it is because a grouping of reaction-patterns is found but, as previously pointed out, the relatively normal personality is difficult to categorize in this way and the psychiatrist's assessment, even if the patient and his friend sustain a miraculous detachment, is highly subjective.

An alternative way of finding out how a patient reacts is to place him in situations and observe his conduct. Insights into the personalities of patients are often obtained by noting how they respond to the standard stress of entering hospital and joining a ward group. Observations of this type are often more reliable than, and always supplement usefully, the data obtained at interview.

Obviously, standardized stresses can be applied to patients by means of psychological tests, the results of which can be expressed without resort to words that carry a load of preconceptions and ambiguity. Objective testing of this kind, corresponding to an extension of the observations of the patient in the ward, can be supplemented by the use of standard questionnaires which, though they leave the patient's subjective bias, can be objectively scored and used for the purposes of comparison with other patients, or with the patient himself at a later stage.

The analysis of test scores on large numbers of patients has shown that certain patterns of scores correlate with certain illnesses. Where distinct personality types are also associated with these illnesses a guess can often be made at the personality characteristic that the tests are measuring. It is hoped that in this way a battery of tests, simple to give and score, will be evolved that can be interpreted to fit familiar verbal descriptions and will at the same time give to the imprecise adjectives a set of operational definitions and a method of quantification.

THE PSYCHOPATH

As previously stated, the psychopath is suffering not only from a personality deviation, but from the disapproval that organized society registers when faced with his behaviour. Definitions of the term psychopath exist by the dozen. A typical example is that of Cheney:

Psychopathic personalities are characterized largely by emotional immaturity or childishness with marked defects of judgement and without evidence of learning by experience. They are prone to impulsive reactions without consideration of others, and to emotional instability with rapid swings from elation to depression, often apparently for trivial causes. Special features in individual psychopaths are prominent criminal traits, moral deficiency, vagabondage, and sexual perversions. Intelligence as shown by standard intelligence tests may be normal or superior, but, on the other hand, not infrequently a border-line intelligence may be present.

This, though one of the best of the definitions, is in reality a compendium of the personality factors that can lead to social difficulties, including the hyperthymic, labile, explosive, and affectionless groupings that Schneider described, together with a list of some of the things of which society disapproves, such as criminality and perversion, in which psychopaths are taken to be prominent participants (if indeed, the implication seems to be, the existence of a criminal or perverted history does not argue that psychopathy is present).

There seems no reason to list, in a definition of psychopathy, the commoner manifestations, except by way of illustration; and it seems less than accurate to link perversions and criminality with psychopathy as it is regarded here, for neither perverts nor criminals are usually psychopaths. Many other similar definitions align themselves alongside the judges by including alcoholics and drug addicts with the psychopaths, but here again, though many psychopaths do take to alcohol or drugs, the majority of addicts are not psychopathic and a large proportion of them probably did not have pre-morbid personality problems of any great consequence before they started to take drugs.

The definition preferred here, that the psychopath is a personality deviant who incurs social disapproval, can be expanded with the aid of some recent work by Cattell on the psychological testing of patients with psychopathic personalities. His group uses letters and numerals to identify traits, thus avoiding the emotional baggage that encumbers the commoner psychiatric terms, but if these are converted to words his findings indicate that the psychopath differs most markedly from normal subjects in that he tends to dominate, to be cheerful and alert but lacking in conscience, and to suffer from excessive tension if frustrated in the expression of instinctual drives. Eysenck's work, using complementary techniques, finds the psychopath slow to condition and to learn.

RESEARCH INTO PSYCHOPATHY

Much of the work done has been vitiated by the imprecision that envelopes the term 'psychopathy', and the double-headed nature of the problem. Research into psychopathy is really research into personality deviation, and research into social nonconformity. These are two separate problems, requiring different training and interests for optimal results in each, and not only might they best be tackled by different psychiatrists, but more accurate work might be done if personality deviation were studied in those untroubled by current social ostracization, and social nonconformity were studied in those uncomplicated by personality deviations. The psychopath is not ideal material for the study of psychopathy.

Nevertheless the hope that psychopathy, regarded inaccurately as a disease, might respond to some form of cure, has led to much optimistic examination of possible causes of the state.

The influence of genes is very important, but is generally ignored because it is impossible, at the present time, to countermand the instructions carried by the genetic codes. The influence of society as it is organized here and now comes in for some attention, but that too is hard to alter, and such evidence as there is does not point to excessively high or low incidence of psychopathy in societies with organizations as different as those found in the U.S.A. and the U.S.S.R.

Environmental influences, particularly in the first few years of life, have been most closely scrutinized, for it is generally believed that such of the personality as is not determined genetically is largely formed under the stimuli of early life. Only controlled work can be more than suggestive, and little of this has been done. It seems, however, that psychopaths have less supervision and parental support as children, together with more public repudiation, though the last may be the consequence of psychopathic conduct rather than its cause. With genetic influences and environmental factors impossible to sort out, it is uncertain whether the poor early circumstances of the psychopathic subjects were the reflection of their parents' abnormal personalities or true causes or both.

It is at this stage in research that the precision claimed for the objective and questionnaire measures of personality traits becomes of the greatest potential use. Clinical observation has determined that certain personality characteristics, such as obsessionality, have a strong genetic basis: obsessionality is known to respond poorly to psychotherapeutic measures. If the separate traits that are genetically decided could be identified, and those moulded by experience determined either by exclusion or experiment, research into childhood influences could be more sharply focused and it would be reasonable to expect that what was formed by environment could be unformed, at least in part, by environmental measures such as intensive psychotherapy.

TREATMENT OF PERSONALITY DEVIATIONS

The use of the word 'treatment' has become conventional in this context: the author wishes to stress that the personality deviations are not necessarily harmful, that even the most severe are not usually the consequence of a pathological process, and that neither psychopathy nor any other personality disorder is an illness. Treatment here means management rather than medication.

Personality deviations as such do not need attention: indeed, statistically abnormal perseverance may be a major asset and gross insensitivity may save much unhappiness.

Personality problems, existing when the patient finds his personality inadequate for the tasks set, are best dealt with by modifying the tasks, since this is so much easier than altering the personality. Where the doctor–patient relationship is authoritarian, the patient may simply be advised to reduce the load; where it is not, he may be educated to know his own capacities and failings. Incidental psychoneurotic reactions (anxiety states, etc.) are dealt with in the usual way, as if they occurred in otherwise normal patients. In certain instances, when factors in the past are thought to be important in the production of the patient's personality and likely to have their late effects modified if properly dealt with, judgements that must be intuitive at our present stage of knowledge, prolonged psychotherapy may be tried.

When the patient is young, and some at least of his personality difficulties resemble those seen in all immature people, prolonged support and educational psychotherapy may be given to tide the patient over a year or two, in the hope and expectation that the passage of time, together with the cumulative effects of a hundred hours of chat, will allow maturation to proceed to the point where the patient needs no more help; it is not easy to know when to stop in these cases, and though it is very helpful for the patient who is improving to be saved from the consequences of previous misdeeds, including the loss of good name that is so hard to recoup, there comes a time with patients who show no signs of improving when the therapy, such as it is, must be terminated and the patient left to learn the hard way.

Psychopaths require treatment as much and as little as other patients with personality problems. They frequently receive it under different conditions, for administrative action or its threat often lies at the back of the original consultation with the psychiatrist. The separation of psychopaths from the normal criminal in certain penal systems has led to the crystallization of useful techniques of management. The general trend today is towards group discussion and participation, with simple and sensible institutional rules which ideally are the fruit of democratic decision by the psychopaths themselves. These techniques are used with profit in criminal institutions such as Herstedvester in Denmark and the Pantucket Institute in Illinois – details and theoretical orientation varying from place to place – and in a few units for personality disorders in psychiatric hospitals. The recent opening of Grendon Underwood, a prison-hospital of the maximum security type, indicates that Britain intends to undertake both research and treatment with the extreme variants to be found among psychopathic criminals, while the psychopaths who are transferred to Broadmoor from the country's prisons show much less disturbed behaviour under the medical régime they encounter there, though some display a certain nostalgia for the jails they left.

dependence
tolerance
withdrawal symptoms } *addiction*

9   Addiction to Drugs

The term addiction is used in medicine in a more restricted sense than is customary in everyday speech, and means more than a liking for a drug or the development of a simple habit. Addiction is said to exist when the patient not only shows psychological dependence (that is to say, expresses and demonstrates his desire to have the drug, using it as a kind of prop) but comes gradually to need increasing quantities of the drug in order to obtain the original effects, and when stopping or severely curtailing the drug is followed by a specific illness called the withdrawal syndrome. These three stigmata of addiction – dependence, tolerance, and withdrawal symptoms – are seen at their most dramatic in the case of heroin, morphine, and allied drugs obtained from raw opium; they are also fairly well demonstrated in alcohol addiction and may be seen, though less commonly, when vulnerable patients have received high dosages of barbiturates or meprobamate for long periods of time.

But addiction is more complicated than this brief introductory statement indicates. If the histories of addicts to various drugs are examined it is found that of the patients who took heroin or morphine for a period of time almost all became addicted; of the subjects who took large doses of alcohol for a long period, less than 5 per cent became addicted; of barbiturate users, a very small proportion ended as addicts. In the case of heroin, morphine, and allied drugs, the predisposition to addiction must be regarded as almost universal, and the problem mainly consists of determining what types of personality reach out for the drugs in the first place, and in what social settings the drugs will be illicitly made available. With alcohol, since for all practical purposes the predisposition to addiction may be regarded as limited to 5 per cent of the population, the problems posed include not only those of personality and social influences but the factors that make one heavy drinker become addicted while nineteen others of apparently equal will-power and demonstrably equal intake do not.

It will be seen, then, that any study of addiction must cover the personality factors of the potential addicts, the social factors conducive to addiction, and in the case of alcohol the individual peculiarities (not necessarily of personality) that mark out some unfortunates as addiction-prone and others as not.

Addiction to morphine, heroin, and other similar drugs is one of the most pitiable conditions seen in medicine, the more so because of the patient's participation in causing the condition he ultimately deplores. The addict attempts to maintain himself in equilibrium by taking adequate doses at set intervals, not disdaining the orgasmic kick associated with intravenous administration of the drug but aiming mainly at the avoidance of withdrawal symptoms. Because of the difficulty of obtaining supplies of drugs equal to the demands of his rising tolerance, and because of a tendency to overspend his stock when it is plentiful, the addict may frequently find himself forced to rub along on inadequate dosages. Though examples do exist of patients who have continued to take the same daily dosage of morphine for years on end, the rule is that larger quantities are needed with time, and that these heavy doses produce complications and side-effects that contribute further to the addict's misery. Once the addict becomes aware of his deterioration he may make serious, even desperate, attempts to break himself of the habit or at least reduce his daily intake. These attempts founder on the withdrawal symptoms, which render the patient frantic with misery and pain and induce as part of the symptom-complex strongly purposive attempts to obtain and administer the drug. At this stage of drug-taking, that of true addiction, the drug has taken on the role of a biological necessity and the patient will exert himself with great vigour and, if need be, unscrupulousness to obtain a supply, no matter how firm his intentions of abstaining before the withdrawal syndrome developed. The patient, in the picturesque jargon, is hooked.

With drugs such as morphine and heroin, most if not all of those who take them or are given them regularly become tolerant and liable to develop withdrawal symptoms. This knowledge should be widespread, and since these drugs should only be obtainable through physicians (who are careful, perhaps over-careful, about inflicting addiction on their patients), the intriguing problem is why addiction should occur at all: the potential addict presumably does not usually intend that he should finish up a suppliant ruin, but he goes to the trouble of taking drugs illegally whose dark reputation he knows and of whose great expense he can hardly be unaware.

The prevention problem is partly one of education. Probably the educated person over-estimates the knowledge that young persons have of the derivatives of opium, and it may be that the inevitability of addiction to these drugs, once they have been used regularly, should be more convincingly publicized.

Unfortunately, though enough is said about heroin and morphine to reach the ears of most young people in the larger towns, the credibility of what is said is often vitiated by the inclusion of the drug called hemp (an ingredient of reefers, also called 'tea' or marijuana) in the list of drugs named as dangerous and addictive. This is inaccurate, since hemp is not addictive and on the whole provides a pleasant and interesting experience that may be regarded as well worth while by its adherents. If a user of hemp finds that he does not feel a need for the drug, that even after long and regular usage he does not have to increase the dose, and that cessation of the indulgence does not lead to withdrawal symptoms, he may wonder if what he has heard about morphine and heroin is really true or, optimistically, whether, though generally true, it applies to him in particular. From the legal and social point of view he has already cast adrift by taking hemp, since this drug seems to be regarded by the judiciary as on a par with the opiates, and turning experimentally to morphine may seem to him a small enough step, large though the difference will later turn out to be. Prejudices against drugs other than alcohol are too ingrained for it to be reasonable to expect that hemp will be freed from the restrictions on narcotics in general, and it may be that its disadvantages, such as they are, are too great for this to be advisable. But it might be helpful if it were not lumped with heroin and morphine in pronouncements from the Bench on its addictive dangers: the young hemp-user who knows better may think that those who warn him against morphine are as wrong, and pay dearly for the assumption.

Prevention would be easier if we knew who was more likely to become addicted. With morphine and allied drugs, as distinct from alcohol, the predilection to addiction is so uniform that the problem resolves itself into the question of who is liable to take morphine in the first place. The first large group of opiate-addicts that may be distinguished are members of the medical and para-medical professions. Doctors, nurses, and pharmacists all have access to these drugs, and the relatively high rate of addiction in this section of the community is eloquent argument for maintaining restrictions on the freedom with which the drugs may be obtained. There are a few addicts who become so because of long and ill-advised courses of morphine or a similar drug administered under medical care; of the few who do start their addiction in this way, most have disordered personalities, though this does not excuse the original mismanagement, since the personality of the patient must be one of the factors weighed when deciding on the propriety of continuing the use of these dangerous drugs for more than a short period.

The rest of the addicts cannot be described as a whole unless the nation harbouring them is specified; in Great Britain, where addiction is rare and drugs are shunned not only by law-abiding citizens but by most of the criminal classes, the personality of the addict is usually highly abnormal; in the United States, where opportunities for obtaining drugs are more frequent in the great cities and the problem is more common and widespread, a less abnormal group may be found, though even here the proportion of gross psychopathy is high; in Chinese quarters where opium-smoking, the least malignant of the types of opiate-intake, is customarily done, the devotees may be normal in their personality make-up. It will be seen that the more the drug is frowned upon and the more difficult it is to get, the more frequently does addiction occur among subjects whose personalities lie outside the normal range.

The most potent determinant of the frequency of drug-addiction is, however, the extent to which commercial interests are concerned. In the larger towns and cities of the United States the narcotics business is run on highly organized lines, and the best principles of commercial and selling organization are mobilized to expand the trade. The pedlars and pushers are assisted by the special property of the opiates, which relieves them of the need to advertise.

By operating a system whereby the drugs are pushed by addicts who receive their own drugs free so long as they can introduce new addicts by a process parallel to seduction, the wholesalers ensure that a large and enthusiastic market is in a state of continual creation. The high prices of drugs obtained illegally make it hard for the addict to keep himself fully medicated, and some addicts drift into the trade of pushing, many (perhaps the majority) to crime; still others from the United States and Canada have recently removed themselves abroad, notably to Great Britain, where prices are easier and regulations, for those already addicted, less stringent.

The low numbers of addicts in Great Britain (probably less than a thousand) and the high numbers in the United States (approaching 50,000) provide a contrast that is incompletely understood on both sides of the Atlantic, and it cannot be pretended that any new explanation is offered here. However, it is probably not the result of any innate resistance to addiction on the part of the British populace, and it can hardly be the result of any administrative measures brought in after addiction has occurred, such as those concerned with the enumeration of addicts. Its most likely cause is the virtual absence, up to now, of any organized importing and selling concern in Great Britain. The low addiction incidence may not continue if closer communion with the continent of Europe allows the Italian influences that are so important in the narcotics racket in the United States to infiltrate across the Channel.

The treatment of established addiction of any kind must

include, whatever preliminary or concurrent psychotherapeutic or other measures are undertaken, total withdrawal of the drug. At one time this was mostly done, in hospitals and prisons, by the abrupt method known, because of the feel and appearance of the addict's skin when the withdrawal symptoms started, as the 'cold-turkey' treatment. Sudden cessation of the drug in this way led to the full flowering of the withdrawal syndrome, with twitching, restlessness, diarrhoea, painful cramps, and abject and miserable pleadings for resumption of the drug. There is no purpose, other than a covertly punitive one, in imposing so miserable a sequence on the patient, and nowadays a more gradual withdrawal, with partial replacement of the opiate by a less potent synthetic drug and the use of sedatives, is the rule. Even with these aids, the ordeal is memorable.

After a week or so the acute craving for the drug subsides, but it is some six months before well-being returns, and the usual recommendation at such experimental centres as Lexington, Kentucky, is that the patient should remain in hospital for at least four months. While the patient stays, he should be investigated to find out, if possible, whether aspects of his life-situation and personality together with any coexisting psychiatric illness may be modified so as to reduce his chances of returning to the addiction after discharge.

In Great Britain and other countries where drugs may only be illicitly obtained in the largest cities, the patient must be persuaded, if possible, not to return to these areas. If the patient is in a medical or one of the auxiliary professions steps must be taken to keep him away from these drugs, if necessary (with the patient's agreement) enlisting the support of his colleagues. Even if all these steps are conscientiously taken and the best attention is unstintingly given, less than one patient in three abstains when he leaves hospital.

This success-rate would be considered poor even if the illness were one of the great plagues such as cholera and the time were the eighteenth century: in these days of potent treatments it is deplorable, and needs explanation. It depends partly on the poverty of the personalities of the addicts themselves; many of them must have found in morphine the only ease and comfort they ever knew, and it is almost impossible to persuade such a person to give up so highly-rewarded an activity as 'main-lining' (administering intravenously) the narcotic of his choice, particularly after a period of abstinence in hospital has made him more susceptible to the pleasant effects of the drug; it is not easy to see how it will ever be done. If the traits in the addict's personality can be analysed and those implicated in his predilection for addiction pin-pointed (in itself no mean task), the exercise is still likely to be one of academic research rather than practical usefulness for the individual concerned; only one method of treatment, psychoanalysis, claims to be able to refashion the personality, and this treatment, even if experimental evidence supported the claims of its enthusiasts, is inapplicable to the dull, the inadequate, the ill-educated, the uncooperative and, in countries where medical attention must be paid for, the poor – adjectives that describe the great majority of the addicts treated. Attempts to persuade patients to keep away from the source of the drugs may fail because the patient cannot earn if he does so, that is if he is a doctor or pharmacist, or because the source seeks him out as part of the service provided by the supply organization. And lastly, the treatment fails because the nature of addiction – the changes that take place at a cellular level and convert the drug from desirable to essential – are not known.

Improvements in the treatment of established addiction to the derivatives of opium and synthetic analogues must come principally from an increase in the knowledge of the intimate biochemical effects of these agents. The addictive process as it appears in alcoholism will be discussed in the next chapter. The main weight of the treatment effort in this disease, as in any other that cannot specifically be eradicated once it has developed but of which the antecedents are known, falls on prophylaxis – prevention is better than cure, the more so when cure is unlikely.

Prevention is undertaken on an international scale by the Commission on Narcotic Drugs of the United Nations Economic and Social Council, which carries on work formerly controlled by the League of Nations. The regulations governing the production and distribution of opium derivatives and of cocaine come under the scrutiny of this body, and the export and import of all narcotic drugs are closely supervised. Unfortunately cultivation of poppies goes on in the Middle East to a greater extent than is necessary to supply legitimate markets, and the excess is diverted to illicit traffic via southern Europe; while in the Far East, where there are hundreds of thousands of addicts, the opium poppy is also widely grown. So long as large areas of poppy-growing continue in countries where the standards of living and therefore of honesty are low the source of the principal drugs of addiction cannot be completely controlled by legislative and administrative measures.

Of the other drugs a few, such as cocaine, are rarely used in medicine today and are therefore less often found to lead to addiction. Most of the others are abused by those patients whose psychological needs predispose them to do so, the drugs themselves – dextroamphetamine, barbiturates, etc. – being comparatively innocuous and easy to obtain by the use of a little dishonest ingenuity.

Dextroamphetamine (dexedrine) is a cerebral stimulant and is one of the few drugs that genuinely increases awareness and some aspects of performance. This drug, as a constituent of Benzedrine, was used in theatrical and other circles during the nineteen-thirties, and its enhancement of wakefulness was exploited by the military during the Second World War. For a long time the drug could be obtained fairly readily, if not in tablet form then as a nasal inhaler from which the active agent could easily be extracted. The stimulant, and some said, the aphrodisiac effects of the drug led to its misuse by certain groups and it became necessary to control its distribution more closely. In Japan it was sold freely for several years after the war and was widely abused by young people catching up on occidental practices.

Though the daily dosage taken by a *habitué* may be as much as two hundred times the standard therapeutic dose, the withdrawal syndrome is mild, usually consisting of no more than slight drowsiness and a tendency to put on weight. This drug is sometimes prescribed to make slimming more easy for women who wish to lose weight without experiencing hunger or feeling

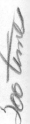

tired because its effects, the reverse of those seen on withdrawal, include increased energy and loss of appetite. Unfortunately, despite the day-dreams of the obese, the boomerang effect of stopping the drug often wipes out the results achieved and the stark fact that weight cannot be lost without feeling hungry or gained without overeating must once again be faced. The advisability of using the drug to assist slimming has been questioned: the fat woman who cannot forgo her carbohydrate is not infrequently using food to deal with a metaphorical emotional starvation, a problem to which dexedrine may come to provide an alternative but even less satisfactory answer.

Apart from the risk of developing habituation, this drug, in common with other cerebral stimulants like phenmetrazine (Preludin) may lead to a psychotic state of great theoretical interest. Readers will remember that the informed speculations about a possible biochemical causation of schizophrenia were many of them concerned with the role of adrenaline and its breakdown products. Dextroamphetamine is chemically and in some ways pharmacologically similar to adrenaline, and its prolonged and excessive use may result in an illness that is clinically indistinguishable from paranoid schizophrenia (though like most psychoses with a known precipitant the outlook is better than that found in the naturally occurring disease). This psychotic state persists long after the drug has left the patient's system and must represent a profound disorder of function resulting from some other factor than the drug's overt pharmacological action.

Barbiturates and other drugs reducing the level of anxiety are used both to induce sleep and to render the tense patient more comfortable and efficient when awake. Barbiturates of one form or another are very widely used, and the rarity of reports of true addiction, as distinct from the habitual use of a mild sleeping capsule, testifies to the safety of this sedative. Most types of insomnia, apart from that found in aged patients, are easily dealt with by the administration of these drugs, which are often continued for years without the dosage creeping up. When the barbiturates are used to blunt anxiety-responses their long-term use is less successful. Anxiety is a reflection of increased awareness and the organism set at a given level of awareness will usually adjust the setting to a higher level if sedative drugs are consistently used, so that higher dosages have to be taken and the risk of addiction becomes real. Probably no sedative drug known at the present time is without addictive risk. The newer sedatives have risks of their own simply because they have not been tested for so many years as the barbiturates, and drugs such as amylobarbitone (Amytal) have not yet been supplanted by newer anxiety-reducing medications.

The conservatism of psychiatrists in this areas has been confirmed or increased by the thalidomide tragedies so widely reported throughout Europe in the early nineteen-sixties. If a patient does become addicted to barbiturates the condition somewhat resembles that seen in alcoholism, a similarity accounted for by the equivalence of the pharmacological actions of the two drugs. The withdrawal syndrome in particular may be indistinguishable from *delirium tremens*, the classical response shown by the alcoholic to sudden termination of his intake or an excessively prolonged bout.

Many other drugs used for therapeutic or experimental purposes have main or side-effects that provide the bored, the curious, or the unhappy with welcome or interesting sensations. The use of hemp has already been mentioned. Mescaline and lysergic acid (L.S.D.), together with other so-called hallucinogens, produce in suitable subjects a fascinating though sometimes alarming psychotic condition which includes in its manifestations hallucinations, illusions, distorted colour, space, and time perception, and sometimes a phenomenon called synaesthesia, meaning the transfer of one kind of sensation to another modality (so that the sound of a violin may induce reddish-brown hallucinations, or the sight of blue steel may cause a cold sensation to spread over the skin). These drugs produce no immediate gratification and are cumbersome to take, so that cases of addiction have not been reported.

Cigarette-smoking, though seldom curiously considered as a form of addiction, is worth mentioning because logically it falls within the addictive group of activities. Heavy, inhaling smokers do develop dependence on cigarettes; they show tolerance, needing to smoke more as time goes by; and they show a comparatively mild but definite and predictable withdrawal syndrome that includes not only the restless seeking of tobacco with associated irritability and abdominal pangs, but changes in the pulse-rate and blood-pressure. Many who frown on addicts are themselves addicted, then, if they regularly take tobacco, particularly in the form of cigarettes. Attention is focused on this form of addiction by the recent official acceptance of long-established data about the enormously increased lung-cancer risks among cigarette smokers. Obviously, psychiatrists can do as little for established cigarette-smokers as they can for heroin addicts; the problem is one of prevention and, therefore, if lessons can be drawn from the history of alcoholism, progressively increasing taxation.

good spirit among canals

10   Alcoholism

Ethyl alcohol is the active constituent of all the intoxicating beverages used in the civilized world. It is consumed in enormous quantities, and though the proportion of subjects who become addicted is small the absolute numbers who take alcohol are so large that alcoholism constitutes a public health problem far more formidable than that posed by any of the drugs mentioned in the last chapter.

The welcome acute effects of alcohol are well known: the subjective feeling of relaxation and warmth, reduction in inhibition, euphoria, camaraderie, and many other consequences of a moderate dose are socially useful and personally pleasant. Personal enjoyment may persist after the social advantages have been nullified by exaggeration – when relaxation turns to inertia, reduction in inhibition to tactlessness and debauch, and the comradely cheer to sentimental loquacity. Even the personal enjoyment may not survive the next morning, when headache, tremulousness, nausea, and lethargy may combine to produce a degree of malaise that is otherwise seldom experienced in the absence of severe illness.

In pharmacological terms these actions of alcohol correspond to the gradual administration of a general anaesthetic. At first the highest functions and the most recently acquired behaviour patterns are impaired – fineness of judgement is reduced, and the accent of origin comes to the fore. Later the capacity to attend to intellectual promptings may become subordinated to emotional pressures which the alcohol discloses – the inebriate may undertake activities that he usually avoids as impolitic and detrimental to his public image, or indulge in easy tears or laughter. Still later the increasingly drunk subject may lose much of the control he commonly exerts, and indulge in instinctual activities of fighting or sexual promiscuity and display, entering a stage corresponding to one seen in anaesthetic induction just before the patient loses consciousness. In a like manner, the next phase for the drunk is that of passing out.

In spite of popular usage, and the evidence of increased activity shown under the influence of alcohol, this drug is not pharmacologically a stimulant. The subject who takes alcohol may feel stimulated, and may believe that his abilities are enhanced, but the true effect of the drug, as demonstrated by objective tests of performance, is one of progressive impairment of intellectual function. The pharmacological explanation of the hangover is rather incomplete: some of the effects are the reverse of the actions of alcohol, notably anxious irritability, while others may be the result of lowered blood sugar.

Alcohol is used not only as a drug, but a food. Its qualifications for inclusion in the honourable category of foodstuffs have been contested, but it is undoubtedly true that at one time citizens of all classes used to obtain a significant proportion of their calories from alcohol, the eighteenth-century boarders at Christ's Hospital School, for example, receiving nearly 40 per cent of their calorific intake from beer. Once alcohol is absorbed it is incorporated into carbohydrate metabolism and may provide energy for the usual activities of locomotion and maintenance of body temperature: it may even indirectly fuel the intellectual activity which in its role as a pharmacological depressant it inhibits.

The normal social and personal effects of alcohol taken in moderation, or occasional excess, whether pleasant or unfortunate, are not usually a medical affair. The doctor enters this scene only because the man who drinks is likely also to drive and may from time to time, whether because he is involved in an accident, has attracted the attention of the police by his erratic progress, or has simply been given a routine check, come into contact with the law. On these occasions the motorist may feel that his driving was normal or even better than his normal, and may be correspondingly indignant. In fact, because of the pharmacological effects of the drug, its presence in the body of a normal person is invariably associated with a decrease in driving skill. The law recognizes that this is so, and that therefore the other users of the highway, who are already risking enough from the everyday hazards of motor traffic, are subjected to an unreasonable chance of injury. Because the injuries sustained may be severe or fatal, and because of the self-induced nature of the driver's disability, the penalties for drunken driving are theoretically severe, and the legislature indicates from time to time its wishes that the maximum penalties should be more frequently imposed.

Nevertheless, as casual observation in the late evening shows, drunk driving goes on and remains largely unpunished. In part, tolerance depends on prevalence: a driver who is punished because his wheels waver as he drives home from the bar is punished capriciously and if the penalty is severe it must seem inequitable. Even the obviously intoxicated driver may be difficult to bring to book, and if he is experienced either in the law or drunkenness it may be almost impossible to obtain a conviction. This is because the driver whose drunkenness is alleged may call on medical opinions of his own choosing: he may also – and if he is wise, will – elect to be tried by a jury, many of whose members will themselves have driven after more alcohol than was prudent. In a trial, and particularly a jury trial, the accused will be given the benefit of any doubt that his witnesses can throw on the case after the prosecution, and if the penalties for the offence are regarded by the jury as unreasonably heavy they will lean over backwards to acquit.

Obviously, what is needed is an objective test of drunkenness that both prosecution and defence can trust. One measure that has been proposed and fairly widely adopted is the introduction of testimony about blood-alcohol level, or some approximation to this derived from the analysis of the subject's exhaled breath. Drawbacks of this type of assay are many, not the least being the human tendency to regard figures written down in black and white as evidence of special worth and dependability. Common experience shows that even among inexperienced drinkers the ability to act in a normal manner after drinking varies widely. The experienced drinker develops a degree of tolerance enabling him to take up to three times as much alcohol as once he could before intoxication becomes apparent. The man who has been drinking for some time also learns to mask his drunkenness, developing a certain skill at behaving staidly when soused; and, more important from the viewpoint of other road users, may have learnt through past frights to modify his driving speeds after he has spent an alcoholic evening. It follows that a blood-alcohol reading is a poor guide to the degree of functional deterioration that a patient will show. Because of the enormous variation in sober-driving skill it is an even less reliable demonstration of the likelihood that driving performance was below standard at the time of the alleged offence. A good driver with great experience of drinking and the kind of nervous system that does not show much lessening of control after ordinary doses of alcohol may drive home after a half-bottle of wine and a large brandy without any feeling of incompetence or guilt; in Sweden, though he drove faultlessly, he would, if apprehended, go to jail.

In the United States evidence of the driver's blood-alcohol is introduced regularly, but does not of itself always constitute complete proof of the accused's state at the time he was charged. The Uniform Vehicle Code Model Chemistry Test Law, which is on the statute books of most of the states of the Union provides that if the driver's blood-alcohol is less than 50 mg. per cent he is deemed sober, if over 150 mg. per cent he is reckoned drunk, and if the assay finds an intermediate figure other evidence must be enlisted to determine the subject's guilt. This law probably allows a few drivers of doubtful sober skill and low capacity for alcohol to get off though they had been driving poorly as a consequence of alcohol; it may also cause the occasional conviction of a subject of high alcohol capacity and considerable driving skill when at the time in question his driving standards were within normal range; though in truth few drivers with a blood-alcohol level of more than 150 mg. per cent can deal properly with novel and alarming situations no matter how smooth and competent their steering and gear-changing may seem in quiet streets. The law's forensic flaw is that it leaves undecided the majority of those cases to which it is applied; however, in a branch of the law where too many acquittals are brought about in the face of the evidence, it provides extra ammunition for the prosecution.

The justice of the drunk-driving laws of most countries is accepted by most people, at least while they are sober. It is necessary to punish those who drive when drink or drugs have rendered them incapable of doing so. Essentially the law applies to driving skill: if this is retained, no case exists, while if it is not, the case is almost complete. It might be that police evidence of erratic driving should be submitted first, and that if this finding is regarded as proved, the level of the driver's blood-alcohol should be introduced as evidence to guide the judge as to the punishment merited. Some reform of the law is needed because of the frequency and ease with which it is flouted, and probably the direction of the change should be towards closer reference to the driver's performance as a driver rather than more detailed examination of aspects of his state thought likely indirectly to bear upon this. In Great Britain the public's covert antagonism to tightening up the drunk-driving prosecutions may prevent indefinitely the full acceptance of chemical evidence.

ABNORMAL DRINKING

Drinking that, by its immediate or delayed effects, causes clear-cut detriment to the health of the drinker or the happiness and material circumstances of his dependants may be regarded as abnormal. Some of those who drink abnormally in this way are alcohol addicts, but the rest are not: the importance of this distinction, from the medical and moral aspect, will be indicated later. Psychiatrists and all others concerned with the problem of alcoholism are indebted to E. M. Jellinek, the founder of the Yale Center of Alcohol Studies, for his realistic classification of abnormal drinkers, which is followed closely in this account and to which specific reference will occasionally be made.

The abnormal drinkers may be divided into those who can stop if they want to and those, the addicts, who cannot. Only those who are not addicted are suitable targets for temperance propaganda, blame, or exhortation, but the allocation of

responsibility is not as simple as the dichotomy seems to indicate: addiction to alcohol takes some time to develop, so that all
the addicts have been at some stage heavy drinkers who could,
had they so desired or had they realized the necessity, have
stopped before addiction supervened.

The non-addicted abnormal drinker uses alcohol hedonisti-
cally or to combat symptoms. He may be a person too much
given to anxiety or unusually unable to tolerate it, or a man with
an actual illness that causes him psychological unrest or pain.
He may occasionally be a man with a gigantic appetite for
enjoyment, a Falstaff in modern dress, who finds that alcohol
enhances some of his pleasures. These alcoholics look forward
to their drinking and show by their conduct that they depend
upon it, but if circumstances call upon them to do so they can
abstain, and if they do not it is egocentricity rather than addictive abrogation of the will that is to blame. In the United States,
where propaganda and information about alcoholism is vigorously disseminated, this type of alcoholic is regarded by many as
ill. Some of these drinkers certainly use the alcohol to reduce
symptoms arising out of coexisting but independent illness, but
for the most part their disorders are of personality, and their
responsibility for their actions and state cannot be set on one
side. In Great Britain and Europe, where alcoholism is regarded
as more of a sin than a sickness, this self-indulgent type of
drinking is thought by many to be the typical manifestation of
alcoholism, the corollary being that the cure for alcoholism is to
be brought about by the use of will-power; this opinion is only
partially justified, and has in common with the opinion that all
alcoholism is a type of illness the attribute of being too sweeping
to fit the data.

Some of these non-addicted alcoholics will become addicted
in time. Those who display no sign of progressing in this way,
the majority, are designed α alcoholics by Jellinek, who resorts
to the Greek alphabet to avoid introducing new and controversial
terms into a field already crowded with emotionally loaded
words. These alcoholics pose a problem for social workers,
employers, police, and many others, and they may bring
tragedy to their families; but they present only uncommonly to

the doctor or the psychiatrist and when they do it may be only because of the insistence of a figure in their circle – a dominating wife, a magistrate, or a solicitous employer. When they do enlist medical aid, whether willingly or under duress, they provide a considerable problem in diagnosis and treatment.

If a specific disease process, such as a psychoneurosis or a psychosis or some non-psychiatric disorder, is found to be present, the treatment may be comparatively easy and sometimes dramatic in its effect. If circumstances are found that Job could not tolerate or Samson overcome, it may be possible to ameliorate these by advice or administrative measures. Commonly no such factors are found, or if they are found cannot be modified, and the physician is faced with a patient who has learned that he can make himself feel better if he takes alcohol and does not see why he should be deprived of this welcome support. The personalities of these patients vary as widely as those of the populace as a whole, except for the tendency they have to experience and resent both depression and anxiety, a tendency greater in its degree than that found in the average person. For these patients, who show no predilection to addiction but only to psychological dependence, it may be possible to substitute some prop other than alcohol to keep gloom and apprehension away.

In a favourable case, the psychiatrist's interest and support may itself suffice, while rarely the psychiatrist may be lucky enough to discover factors in the patient's past that may be implicated in his present unease, and whose malign influence can be permanently modified by psychotherapy: this treatment would be used with greater success with patients of the non-addicted group if the group as a whole were more highly motivated to cooperate. Sometimes a drug such as one of the barbiturates may be temporarily administered to the patient instead of alcohol, but drugs, no matter how close their pharmacodynamics to those of alcohol, can never provide the incidental benefits of drinking – the warmth, the welcome, the physical escape, and the company of men. It is here that Alcoholics Anonymous can come to the aid of the physician whose therapeutic resources are inadequate: this organization will be described in some detail later in the chapter, when the types of alcoholism have been more fully set out.

Some alcoholics drink heartily and recklessly for many years without coming into more than trivial conflict with organized society. They may have no dependants or do them little disservice – a rather dull and gloomy patient of my acquaintance had a wife and children who, having tried him drunk and sober, on the whole preferred him drunk. A proportion of these patients develop the physical complications of alcoholism, such as cirrhosis of the liver, and present to the doctor in this way. Alcoholic cirrhosis, and many other physical complications, may fail to progress and may improve if alcohol is abandoned, and some of these patients may be induced to give it up by placing emphasis on the evidence of physical disease. In Jellinek's classification non-addicted but physically ill drinkers are designed β alcoholics.

A distinct division may now be drawn between the alcoholics so far described and the *alcohol addicts*. The addicts drink to excess and damage their careers and families like the α alcoholics: they may develop cirrhosis of the liver and thus resemble β alcoholics. But they also show the stigmata of true addiction: not only do they have psychological dependence, but their tolerance rises and they either show withdrawal symptoms on abstention or, in the commoner of the two varieties of addiction, lose control of their intake. How the heavy drinker becomes an alcohol addict, how he progresses from self-indulgence to true illness, may be best illustrated by recounting in detail an imaginary but characteristic history.

A man, perhaps of a lonely and rather sad disposition, finds solace and jovial company in the bar and spends too much of his time and money there, quieting his conscience by small rationalizations or, more frankly, admitting to himself that the money should go to his family and setting his need for pleasure alongside theirs, only to find that his is the greater. At this stage he is not only indistinguishable from an α alcoholic from the outside but he himself, were he asked, would classify himself as belonging to the α group if he admitted that his drinking was excessive at all. If he is destined to become an addict, the first thing he may notice is that his tolerance starts to rise. Where freedom from care was formerly achieved with four drinks, six are now needed. Where an evening with friends who pour small tots was formerly no more than a mild imposition it now becomes positively abhorrent unless some extra drinks can be jocularly elicited or a loading dose is taken before the social evening starts.

The drinker who spends his evenings with like-minded friends whose tolerance is not rising will notice that their rhythm, once matching his, no longer does so: he has to take extra drinks surreptitiously during the evening, or arrive before they do, or leave later. These actions are positive and require planning: they occur outside the activities of the group, and are undertaken with insight. The patient knows from folk-lore what is happening to him, and at this time, for a brief period, may become inclined to seek treatment. If he heeds the warnings of guilt he will find, even at this comparatively embryonic stage, that his alcoholism will be treated primarily by complete and permanent abstention, an interdict that the patient may reject, supposing it punitive or arbitrary.

After a couple of years more the patient, as he has now inevitably become, reaches the 'crucial phase'. Already his reaction to alcohol is showing an abnormal pattern: he may experience what are called palimpsests (meaning parchments that have been wiped clean of writing), when he fails to recall what happened to him on the previous evening *though during the period in question he did not appear drunk*, and his life has come to revolve round alcohol. During the crucial phase he finds himself losing control for the first time: an evening's drinking is prolonged into the night, the patient stopping only when he is too wretched, too broke, or too drunk to continue. These minor 'benders' make the alcoholic angry and ashamed, and are often followed by a resentful contrition and a spell of abstemiousness.

The immediate physical consequences of stopping drinking after a bout may be gratifying, but without alcohol the patient has to look at his life and works without the benefit of his usual blur; the view is often depressing. Also delayed abstinence effects, usually spells of gloom or agitation, start after a few days and drive the patient to rationalize his drinking habits: optimistically, and with many resolutions about restriction of intake, he starts again. Another bout ensues, and misery, remorse, and self-reproach return. It is not part of the pattern of human beings, particularly those depending on alcohol, to blame themselves for long if others are to hand: the alcoholic turns on his family, his friends and his medical advisers. If he is 'on the wagon' he awaits only a slighting word or an action upon which an unfriendly construction can be placed to argue, using the subsequent quarrel as an excuse for returning to the bottle. When drinking he may protect his self-esteem by continuing his paranoid utterances or making gestures that are grandiose in their generosity and expanse or both. An alcoholic acquaintance, who insisted that all the guests at his table at a Hunt Ball should pay for nothing, overriding their protests with such determination that they were forced to agree, turned to me immediately they had consented, to say with tears in his eyes, 'The bastards are bleeding me dry.'

As this phase goes on the alcoholic loses interest in food and his sexual performance starts to fail; the former makes him drink more and reduces his vitamin intake, while the latter, by a psychological process easy enough to understand, makes him suspicious of his wife's morals. This jealousy may be the last straw for a long-suffering wife, and the family structure, if indeed it has lasted this long, starts to disintegrate. The patient's home life collapses about his ears, and he turns, as he has always turned, to more alcohol.

From this time on he deteriorates steadily: he starts drinking in the mornings, eats little, loses his job, moves down the social scale, indulges in longer and more frequent 'benders', and at last, in degraded circumstances, reaches 'rock-bottom'. At this point, when rationalization, man's most powerful defence, can no longer hide his plight and his failure, the chronic alcoholic may at last seek treatment.

This general pattern of the rake's progress is characteristic of the alcoholics of Great Britain and the United States and some other countries where spirits are the commonest form of alcohol used by heavy drinkers. Quantitative variations are seen – men may take twenty years to complete it, while women may come to the end of the line after only three or four years of drunkenness; periods of abstention, undertaken because of the influence of dominant members of the patient's family and with the aid of hospital treatment, or because of administrative measures such as imprisonment, may lengthen the course. Once fully embarked upon, however, the untreated illness is inexorable, so that treatment is essential if a humiliating and uncomfortable end is to be avoided.

In some parts of the world alcoholism shows individual features that differ from those seen in the Anglo-Saxon countries. In Finland, where absolute social conformity is a feature of the culture and alcohol tends to be taken seldom but in large tots of spirits, the drinker may suddenly lose self-control, as if the rapidly rising blood-level of alcohol acted like inhaled ether, and viciously attack his neighbour. The homicide rate, which is higher in Finland than in any other civilized country, consists mainly of murders committed by acutely drunk people.

In France, where wine is all but worshipped and alcohol is regarded as a proof of God's benevolence, a form of alcoholism exists that is seldom seen elsewhere: the rural Frenchman may start his day with a bottle of wine, top up during the morning with hourly glasses, take another bottle at lunch-time, follow on with hourly glasses during the afternoon, and finish off another bottle or two in the evening. This kind of alcoholic, by never appearing drunk, escaped attention for many years. Probably the high incidence of alcoholic cirrhosis in France first focused attention on the problem, but the clinical signs of alcoholism as this is known in the spirit-drinking countries are mostly absent. The French alcoholic does not lose control; he does not usually deteriorate; he does not show withdrawal symptoms because alcohol is, apart from accidents, never withdrawn and it is probable that at no time of day or night does his blood-alcohol level fall to zero. Only if this type of alcoholic falls ill does his latent alcoholism achieve recognition: the illness itself may be the consequence of alcoholism, or it may, by causing alcohol to be withdrawn, give the patient delirium tremens.

The *treatment* of late alcohol addiction is undertaken hopefully in each instance, and unwavering optimism is or should be displayed. The results are humiliatingly bad.

The alcoholic is admitted and all sources of alcohol are cut off. His general health is attended to and vitamins are given because his reduction in food-intake has deprived him of these essential dietary ingredients while his alcohol intake has increased his requirements of them. If he cannot sleep he is sedated and if he cannot sit or lie still he is given simple tranquillizers. Reassurance and support tide him over the acute manifestations of withdrawal, unless he becomes delirious.

Delirium tremens, the classical consequence of prolonged heavy drinking especially if alcohol is suddenly stopped at a time when the organism is weakened, is heralded by increasing agitation and restlessness, and a nervous apprehension and suspicion that indicate that the patient is ceasing to grasp what is happening around him and is, as a consequence, taking the only safe course in this unfriendly world and assuming that he is being got at. His sleep becomes restless and disturbed by vivid and alarming dreams. His consciousness becomes more clouded and he starts to interpret what he dimly sees and hears in such a way that his perceptions fit his mood, which is often one of apprehensive remorse. Voices, sometimes those of loved ones, reproach him with his misdeeds, and the patient may be hard put to it to explain how the owners of the voices manage to hide in his bare room without showing themselves. Visual hallucinations, often starting on an illusional basis, say from a crack in the wall, cause the patient's fear to increase to the point where he may cry out or attempt to run away. He may see small animals, or complex scenes; snakes, rats, insects, and all manner of horrid things (but not, in practice, pink elephants) may emerge from the floor and converge upon him, or soldiers may march and counter-march on the bed-table, with brass bands playing.

These phenomena grip the patient in fearful fascination, but are seldom so enthralling that he cannot be distracted, at least for a time, by stimuli from the real world. Thus the patient, though he is obviously unpleasantly hallucinated when one enters the room and may believe himself to be incarcerated in a zoo or back at his work as a tic-tac man, lorry driver, or surgeon, will usually answer questions and temporarily grasp the necessity of submitting to medical procedures: reassurance, though gratefully accepted, is of fleeting value, for once the real stimuli stop or by continuing lose their novelty the patient is drawn back into his delirious perceptions.

Delirium tremens, the subject of scores of jokes and stories, is a dangerous illness. At one time one patient in six died, and a proportion of the survivors failed to recover their intellectual powers. Even at present an occasional patient may die or show dementia, but the mortality and morbidity have been reduced by modern treatments. The delirium itself is controllable to some extent by phenothiazine drugs: with the help of these and sedatives (not barbiturates) at night, the episode is made less exhausting and the hallucinatory experiences may be shortened or rendered less vivid. In many instances death and dementia used to come not from the direct effects of alcohol or even from the immediate consequences of taxing delirium, but from vitamin deficiency; today vitamin deficiency is rare if a normal diet is taken. Treatment with massive doses of vitamins is resorted to at an early stage of the treatment of alcoholism and may prevent the onset of delirium or abort its course; even if it does not shorten the episode, it reduces the overall mortality and prevents the complications (Korsakoff's syndrome and Wernicke's encephalopathy), that used not uncommonly to emerge as the delirium ceased.

Once the patient has recovered from the acute effects of alcohol withdrawal he is often surprised at the ease with which he can accustom himself to a day without alcohol. As little as forty-eight hours after stopping drinking the patient may find that his shakiness has started to diminish, his appetite is increased, and his craving for alcohol, though he would not refuse a drink if it were pressed upon him, is gone. This is so different from his previous experiences when he tried to modify his intake on his own and so unlike his apprehension at the time of admission that the patient frequently feels a surge of optimism and confidence and may think of discharging himself to return to his work and family. Sometimes patients actually take their leave, in which case arrangements may confidently be made for their readmission.

Withdrawal, as such, is the easy part. It is the long siege that follows that claims the casualties. Perhaps more than most human beings, the alcoholic is better able to stand a short sharp dramatic tussle than a long and boring war. After the subsidence of acute restlessness and craving the patient is faced with what amounts to a specific illness – called by M. Wellman the late withdrawal symptoms. The patient feels free from craving for alcohol, but becomes irritable and depressed; his sleep is broken, he tires easily and his concentration is poor. It is natural for him to believe himself one drink below par, and for six months or so he may seldom feel as well as he did during the early stages of his alcoholism when his alcohol level was at a subjective optimum, and though he still probably feels better than he did during the phase of alcoholism that existed immediately before his admission it is for the first drinking years rather than the last that the brooding, depressed, and abstinent alcoholic yearns. Not until a year or eighteen months have passed does the alcoholic find that the patches of depression start to lessen to the point where they become tolerable and controllable, and until this time he is severely at risk: it is all too easy for him to return to drink to reduce his symptoms, perhaps, or to forget a domestic quarrel into which his irritability has led him as surely as once his projected guilt used to.

It is obviously out of the question that the patient should spend eighteen months, or even the high-risk first six months, in hospital; few individuals could pay for such a stint and no community could underwrite such prodigal expenditure for its alcoholics. Much of the research effort in alcoholism is directed at finding ways in which the alcoholic may be protected from his tendency to start drinking again shortly after he leaves hospital. In this respect psychotherapy directed against the patient's personality defects, even if successful beyond all hopes, is not the complete answer: the remodelled personality will still belong to an addict, and the addict will still suffer from the near-intolerable blues and reds of the late withdrawal syndrome. This difficult period is treated in several ways, all of them designed to prevent the alcoholic taking his first drink. An absolute embargo on alcohol is laid down because once an abnormal addictive drinking pattern has been established it will recur with astonishing speed after drinking is resumed, even though a long period of abstinence may have intervened; also it is my impression that even a brief lapse can put off the time when well-being returns by a disproportionate period.

The psychotherapeutic method consists of exhortation of greater or lesser subtlety. The patient is told with absolute certainty that his days of drinking are over, and that he can never be a social drinker again. His attempts to show how his pleasure in company and the company's pleasure in him will diminish, or how a few drinks are essential to the smooth running of his business are countered by examples of people and groups who lead pleasant and sociable lives or succeed at business without drinking. His genuine embarrassment at the prospect of having to refuse a drink is diminished by assurance that this can successfully be done, and perhaps by mentioning, as possible excuses he can proffer, the illnesses that may be contracted perfectly respectably and yet prevent the convalescent from taking alcohol, notably jaundice.

The patient, thinking along the obvious lines of will-power and courage, and ignoring the lessons his own illness should have taught him, will most commonly jib at the prospect of a lifetime without a drink. At a bleak time of life he sees nothing but a bleak prospect ahead of him, and is unlikely, no matter how good his relationship with his doctor, to make much of the medical prediction that in a year or so he will feel much better. Sometimes the patient who remains unconvinced will respond to the information that many alcoholics do not believe that alcohol must be for ever avoided and that it often takes two or three innings before such few as survive will acquiesce. During this prolonged attempt to get the addict to face facts and realize that abstention is not some temperance fad but a medical essential, other less important habits of thought may be encountered. The patient will frequently express remorse about the way he has treated his family and friends, but often his phraseology is as grandiose and as suspect as that which he once used about his successes when fully alcoholized and in congenial company: this does not necessarily reflect real insincerity on the patient's part – he may have started drinking to get away from or to spite a spouse who gave him only the edge of her tongue, and now, though he feels she has suffered too much, nevertheless thinks that she would have been too lucky had she got off scot-free.

If these resentments are brought out into the open realistic aims may be more easily defined: all that may still be possible is that the patient can support his family, quieting his conscience but applying no balm to his soul. Over the whole psychotherapeutic course, it is important to preserve the patient's dignity: the whole treatment programme is wounding and its resemblance to punishment, which is accidental but striking, must be explained to the patient's satisfaction. This task is not easy, but is seldom a hardship; many alcoholics are most likeable and not simply because of their typical (but not universal) easy *bonhomie*; often the factors that led them to alcohol are productive of great sympathy and their ultimate plight, with so many reminders of early promise still apparent, most pitiful. This simple type of psychotherapy must be continued after the patient leaves hospital, perhaps for years; if his family is still congenial and cooperative after their trials and disappointments they can be of great assistance, provided that they too grasp the necessity for total abstention. Here again, Alcoholics Anonymous may help the physician out by providing what he cannot – the constantly available support and companionship of men who have themselves been through the mill.

The waves of depression and agitation, resembling in magnification the feelings of a man whose regular evening meal is delayed and perhaps depending on a similar mechanism, may come upon the patient suddenly and, especially during the first few months, be severe and long-lasting enough to make his work and social relationships suffer. Even if he has been warned in detail of these bouts, the patient cannot be expected to deal with them unaided. Sometimes the alcoholic may be able to weather each storm by calling on the help of a fellow A.A. member, but many patients will benefit from the use of drugs. Physicians are naturally hesitant to use fresh anxiety-reducing drugs on patients who have just been weaned from such a drug, and A.A. literature specifically warns alcoholics off props of this kind. However, the occasional use of drugs under medical supervision does not seem to delay the time when these episodes of tension and gloom start to wane, and the patient is unlikely, over such a short period, to become more than mildly habituated even if he resorts to the sedatives with unusual regularity.

Probably some alcoholics, those whose personalities are such that they tolerate discomfort very poorly, are unsuitable for sedation while others, those whose addictive pattern of drinking arose out of needs other than symptomatic relief, may take them for a while with impunity: in the safe and popular phrase, each case must be judged on its merits. The recently developed anti-depressive drugs, to which addiction has not been reported, may be recommended, and in time will probably cause A.A. and other antagonists of drug therapy in alcoholism to withdraw in part their sweeping objections.

The measures so far described for the alcohol addict in remission are useful and necessary. They still are unlikely, used alone, to prevent the alcoholic from trying just one drink at a time when confidence or misery warp his judgement or the words of old and resentful companions sting him into proving his manhood. Physicians aim, somehow or another, to take the pleasure out of the thoughts of the first drink. Clumsily, they do so by substituting nausea or fear.

Aversion treatment, the most common application of pure Pavlovian conditioning techniques to medical treatment, aims at inducing in the patient a feeling of nausea when he contemplates a drink. It is an abhorrent and disgusting procedure. A typical régime causes the patient to be placed in a featureless room without natural lighting, there to lie until by his response to proffered alcohol he is judged 'averse'. Every two hours, on the hour, the patient is given an injection of a potent emetic such as apomorphine. This enters the blood-stream and, when it reaches the appropriate 'trigger-zone' of the brain, induces nausea and retching in the patient. The time that this takes to happen is soon found by experience, and just before the nausea supervenes the patient is offered an alcoholic beverage. As he gulps it the nausea starts and increases, and as soon as he has vomited it another drink, usually the patient's favourite but sometimes another to cover the range commercially obtainable, is pressed upon him. When the nausea diminishes the exhausted patient is allowed to rest.

Two hours later, the same process starts again, and as the days and the indistinguishable nights go by the bottles and the vomitus, which are not taken away, give to the room an air of almost unmatchable squalor. Sooner or later the patient starts to puke at the mere sight of a glass or the sound of a bottle-opener; he tries to swallow but cannot; he weakly pushes the glass away. By these and other signs, best not published, the attending doctor is able to recognize that the patient has developed the conditioned reflex of responding to the sight, sound, smell, and taste of alcohol with nausea, and the treatment is at an end after several days of misery.

Some patients back down after lasting only a few hours; others, more conscious of contractual obligations, attempt to feign reflex aversion and end the treatment in that way – one patient, congratulated on finishing his treatment, rashly agreed that it would be pleasant to celebrate the end of the ordeal by joining the doctor in a glass of champagne, and was given a further three days. Most alcoholics last the course, perhaps because they feel, in their remorse, that even if it does not work, even if they secretly intend to return to alcohol, the régime of degradation is no more than they deserve.

While the treatment is going on the patient sometimes becomes very dependent and suggestible, as who would not, and the opportunity may be taken of administering psycho-therapy, not necessarily directly related to alcohol; patients listen attentively to a doctor who apparently believes his words important enough to keep him in an atmosphere which the patient would pay large sums to be removed from, and a thera-peutic relationship may be firmly cemented in the aversion chamber.

The conditioned reflex that is learnt by the patient is, despite the show and the price, a poor and weakly thing; it is contradictory to and much more recent than most of the other conditioned reflexes he has learned in relation to alcohol. Therefore it is easy for patients to overcome the conditioned reflex if they so choose, by drinking regardless of the nausea once they have left hospital until the reflex fades by lack of reinforcement. The treatment is often criticized for this real failing, but its usefulness lies in its assistance to the alcoholic who genuinely does not wish to succumb to temptation. It may, by making him veer away from rather than into a bar-room doorway, be crucial in his cure.

Fear of alcohol as a source of symptoms is sometimes found to occur naturally in the alcohol addict who has taken a long look at himself as he descended the skids. It may have been induced or increased by his physician's matter-of-fact statements about the course of unchecked alcoholism or relapse. But his theoretical, far-sighted, respectful fear is not enough to prevent many alcoholics from taking the easy or what may seem the only way out of a bout of crippling malaise that besets them during that protracted convalescence. A method of preventing the alcoholic from taking drink was discovered by chance in Denmark in 1948. Two research workers who were testing a drug, tetraethylthiuram disulphide (T.E.T.D.), on themselves as part of its preliminary investigation as a treatment for worms, became distressed and ill after taking a small amount of alcohol at a party. They connected this untoward reaction with the T.E.T.D. in their systems, and undertook an examination of the mode of action of the drug.

It was found that T.E.T.D., after absorption and probably after degradation within the body to some other product, alters the metabolism of alcohol: usually alcohol is rapidly degraded through various stages, and the intermediate products are present in such small quantities and for such a short time that their pharmacological properties are of no significance for the organism. T.E.T.D. blocks the metabolism of alcohol at the acetaldehyde level, presumably by interfering with the action of the enzyme that usually prevents the acetaldehyde from existing more than momentarily. When a patient has taken T.E.T.D., then, imbibing alcohol leads to the production, if the drug is working with total effectiveness, of equimolecular quantities of acetaldehyde, a substance that is highly toxic if present in any significant concentration. In effect, if the alcoholic takes alcohol, he poisons himself; even without T.E.T.D. he does that, but with T.E.T.D. he does so immediately and for the alcoholic it is promptness of toxicity rather than severity that is so salutary.

T.E.T.D., known as Disulfiram or by the trade-name Antabuse, is given to the alcoholic in hospital for a few days and then he is given a sample of his usual brand of liquor – preferably, if he is suspicious, from a newly opened bottle. Ten minutes or so after drinking it, which few can do without a reminiscent smile, the patient finds that the warm glow he knows so well is getting out of hand: his face flushes and continues to suffuse until he resembles a turkey and the eyes distend and become bloodshot (the 'bull-eye' or 'ox-eye'); the pulse pressure increases and the patient experiences widespread throbbing and headache; he becomes uneasy, alarmed, and breathless; sweating, nausea, and vomiting increase his fear and discomfort, and even more severe consequences may ensue. At the end of the reaction he may fall into an exhausted sleep, but the full rigours of the experience remain fresh in his memory when he wakes.

Few patients will drink while taking Disulfiram, and it is the knowledge that they cannot do so that makes so many alcoholics reject it on the specious grounds that they want to master the problem unaided. Both this drug and another called Temposil (a similar but milder preparation) will enable the patient to resist alcohol by being strong for two minutes at a time, when he takes the drug, instead of maintaining his resolve throughout the day. If the addict, because of some quarrel or autonomous mood-change, decides that he will start drinking again and stops his Disulfiram, he still has to wait a few days before the drug clears from his system: it gives him a chance to reconsider. If, as some physicians commonly advise, the drug is regularly administered by the spouse, the home atmosphere becomes less tense and apprehensive, for another few days' peace is guaranteed to a household accustomed to being poised endlessly on the brink of fresh disaster.

Unfortunately Disulfiram is not entirely free from side-effects: it often causes patients to complain of minor psychological symptoms, and though these are difficult to sort out from post-alcoholic malaise it is probable that some at least are due to the drug; also it makes taking any alcohol – in a sauce, in a chocolate or even, via the skin, in after-shave lotion – a hazardous procedure and the patient so medicated must take great care that he does not innocently trigger off an acetaldehyde reaction.

After-care once the patient has left hospital is of the greatest importance. It is uncertain how best the addict should be treated, as the low success-rate attests, but support, reassurance, and at least the outward signs of affection should be offered as frequently as need be. If the patient's relationships with his family are relatively good the doctor may enlist the support and progress-reports of the spouse, but this, though desirable, may have to be relinquished if the patient finds the intervention of others demeaning or feels that his status as a patient is being diluted. The intervention of such agencies as the Church, though theoretically welcome, is in practice not always useful: the subject of alcohol addiction is not distinguished clearly in the lay mind from the vice of self-indulgence with which, indeed, it has at one time overlapped in each history; therefore the attitudes of exponents of morality are liable to show ethical disapproval, whereas at this stage the addict is usually all too aware of his guilt and rather than requiring it to be increased needs to put it to one side in order that he may attend to the personal rehabilitation that is his main current aim.

The most hopeful group to whom the patient may be introduced, preferably while he is still in hospital, is Alcoholics Anonymous. This extraordinary organization was founded in the United States just before the Second World War and has increased its membership and geographical spread consistently since then. It was formed by alcoholics and its principles show an intimate knowledge of the alcoholic's plight and patterns of reaction. The group aims only at helping other alcoholics to recover: it extracts no dues and makes no conditions for membership – the alcoholic is automatically a member from the moment the idea of joining enters his head; A.A. has no affiliation to other groups and offers no individual item that is novel, but only a helpful amalgam of old medical and religious saws.

The alcoholic, once he has been to a meeting, is usually caught unless he is too psychopathic or brain-damaged to enter into group activities. He meets other men who have matched or surpassed his drinking and is present at conversations where the general and confident assumption is that those who do not stop drinking after alcoholism supervenes will die or go mad. He sees patients who have got better and look happy and well-fed, and his rationalizations, so successful with gullible friends and relatives, are met with forgiving smiles by men who, if he fumbles for a moment, will helpfully finish his sentences for him. Even if he does not stop drinking there and then the first meeting with A.A. has great impact, and many alcoholics who have cried off at the time they were introduced return when their rationalizations finally fail. To remain dry, the alcoholic may try the Twelve Steps that A.A. suggests: the organization makes it known that these are not inviolate but only apparently useful, and no member is required to subscribe to them; the group is closely knit, however, and most group members adopt part or all of this loose doctrine in order that they may fully share the corporate aims. These Twelve Steps are as follows:

1. We admitted we were powerless over alcohol – that our lives had become unmanageable.
2. Came to believe that a Power greater than ourselves could restore us to sanity.
3. Made a decision to turn our will and our lives over to the care of God as we understood Him.
4. Made a searching and fearless moral inventory of ourselves.
5. Admitted to God, to ourselves, and to another human the exact nature of our wrongs.
6. Were entirely ready to have God remove all these defects of character.
7. Humbly asked Him to remove our shortcomings.
8. Made a list of all persons we had harmed, and became willing to make amends to them all.
9. Made direct amends to such people wherever possible, except when to do so would injure them or others.

10. Continued to take personal inventory and when we were wrong promptly admitted it.
11. Sought through prayer and meditation to improve our conscious contact with God as we understood Him, praying only for knowledge of His will for us and the power to carry that out.
12. Having had a spiritual awakening as the result of these steps, we tried to carry this message to alcoholics and to practise these principles in all our affairs.

These steps read strangely to the worldly and sober European, but they work better than most of the elegantly argued scientific treatments. The alcoholic admits that his drinking is out of control, and he can do so with ease and perseverance because his companions share his knowledge. He sees hope in the group and if only for that reason loses anxiety and becomes ready to embrace whatever credo is offered, much as a patient reacts in any psychotherapeutic situation. The mobilization of God enables the guilt the alcoholic feels to be relieved somewhat, while at the same time he is enjoined and encouraged to make amends when he can to those he has harmed, a process that increases his self-respect as soon as it has begun.

The alcoholic also helps others: from being an object of pity and scorn he finds that he is able to assist those worse off than he. He will do so with skill and expertise because of his own experience, so that he strengthens his own principles and beliefs by subtly preaching them, and gains a spiritual pleasure from helping fellow-sufferers. A.A. literature refers again and again to the fact that these principles, whatever their psychological rationale, work – 'and with us who are on the way to the asylum or the undertaker anything that works looks very, very good indeed'. A.A. estimates that *of those who stay in the organization 50 per cent become abstemious at once, and a further 25 per cent recover after relapses.* Of those three out of five who abandon A.A. after a brief trial many return later when alcoholic damage has done its evangelical work and forced them into an untenable moral and physical position.

The organization of A.A. groups is uniquely informal: Parkinson's Laws do not seem to apply. A.A. groups are all independent, financially and organizationally; they accept no money from outside and express no opinions on outside issues; they maintain personal anonymity at all times; but A.A. groups are not bound to follow these guiding principles, which are merely formulated by a central liaison body, the General Service Office, on the basis of information received about A.A. groups over the world: in an organization where any two alcoholics, meeting by chance and expressing the wish that they could stop drinking, may consider themselves an A.A. group no tight control is possible and to the observer who abhors the dead hand of over-administration it seems that this fluidity and de-centralization is one of the mainsprings of the continuing live-liness and value of Alcoholics Anonymous.

The numbers of A.A. members throughout the world, includ-ing those whose continuing sobriety has led them to allow their attendances to lapse, is about 250,000 and most sizeable towns in Anglo-Saxon countries have one or more branches: evidently, where no branch exists, one may easily be formed, while A.A. will maintain contact with the few members who are so isolated that they can find no other alcoholic in their area.

Alcoholics Anonymous maintains cordial relationships with the medical profession. It sends members who are ill to doctors and cooperates with hospitals where its help is asked for. Yet it was formed because doctors had no cure for alcoholism. Its future, if a cure is discovered, must be modified by this new knowledge. Since A.A. regards alcoholism as a spiritual flaw rather than a medical condition, there exists a possible point of friction if basic knowledge of the addictive process increases: it would be a great pity if A.A. and medical practitioners came to compete for patients because both felt, as now only one group feels, that they had the therapeutic answer.

The crux of the matter is that alcoholism is not one problem but many problems: no one method of treatment is likely to be applicable to all cases. A.A.'s success is mainly with the psycho-therapeutic aspect of the treatment of alcoholism, providing as it does catharsis, conversion, massive group support, and solid friendships; with these patients, particularly non-addicted

alcoholics, whose main subjective gain from alcohol is a semblance of group approval, A.A. is highly successful. With those
patients who are physically or psychiatrically ill or who display the signs of true addiction, formal medical measures are
either already more appropriate or may, when knowledge of
the nature of addiction allows specific treatments to be elaborated, become so. These two categories of patient are not
mutually exclusive, and for the physician A.A. can almost
always provide help and expert inside knowledge. It is to be
hoped that medical measures will shortly be able to offer more
effective help to A.A.

PRESENT TRENDS

Overall, the problem of alcoholism is diminishing throughout
the world, so that claims for the effectiveness of a variety of
public health measures cannot be allowed if they rest only on
evidence of a falling incidence. In certain countries where
complex internal strains exist, such as Poland, the incidence of
alcoholism is still rising, but even from this example it is unwise
to draw facile conclusions for West Germany also had increasing
alcoholism in the post-war years.

The most convincingly successful public health measure ever
carried out was probably Prohibition: the Prohibition era in the
United States is often remembered there and elsewhere as one
of widespread bootlegging and corruption, and though it is true
that the law was widely ignored it is also a fact that the figures
for alcoholism and allied conditions such as cirrhosis showed a
sharp fall while the enactment continued in force. The Prohibition legislation was carried by powerful temperance lobbies and
was so widely disapproved by saner citizens that its full enforce-
ment was impossible; even so it achieved many of the hopes of its
instigators. Because alcoholism, both addictive and non-addic-
tive, is so difficult to treat once it is established – even A.A.
reaches less than 5 per cent of the alcoholics in the United States
– prevention by large-scale administrative measures is the most
promising method.

The temperance (i.e. intemperately abstemious) interests in

Great Britain had much influence in the second half of the nineteenth century and unsuccessfully proposed legislation to restrict the consumption of alcohol: their measures were too fanatical to command support, and may have alienated it in a country self-consciously concerned to avoid statutory prohibitions. Their main immediate success lay in the blue-ribbon movement, those who had taken the pledge (of total abstention) declaring themselves T.T. by a piece of ribbon in the lapel. Ultimately, however, laws to limit the numbers of outlets for liquor were passed (the Licensing Act, 1904) and taxation of alcoholic beverages was progressively increased to the point where, to an Englishman, almost any other country in the world seems to sell cheap drinks. Over this period, for some reason and perhaps for these legislative and price-increasing reasons, the rate of severe alcoholism in Great Britain, once notoriously high, fell to the present rather low rate of about 1:1,000, but it is hard to believe that the general increase in nutrition and living standards did not in some way contribute to the altered habits of drinking.

In the United States the experience with Prohibition has prevented other, milder legislation from being enacted (as the temperance movement in Great Britain, may, by its immoderation, have delayed desirable legislation), and in general in the United States (with an alcohol-addiction rate more than four times as high as ours) alcohol may be obtained both freely and cheaply. In Scandinavian countries, particularly Sweden and Finland, liquor-sales are closely controlled by law. In wine-growing countries, of which France is the most important, the problem of alcoholism is too controversial for a democratically elected legislature to touch, and there is no expectation of restrictive reforms becoming law.

On common-sense grounds it seems likely that with a steady level of national income, and given that food was not excessively expensive, legislation causing the price of alcohol to rise to the point where it was difficult to pay for without cutting into money set aside for essentials and yet not high enough to encourage more than marginal smuggling or illegal distillation, would reduce the number of heavy drinkers and therefore of alcoholics and alcohol addicts. Democracies with special liquor interests exerting pressures on the elected representatives or with distinct cultural biases in favour of alcohol among the electorate may find it difficult to enact laws along these lines: the Communist countries of Eastern Europe, with large alcohol problems and no electorate to worry about, can deal with this aspect of alcoholic prophylaxis more incisively, though their ability to resolve social problems may not be so great.

Propaganda against alcohol is an uncertain method, but one that has possible applications if skilfully done. Propaganda, unfortunately, if directed against undesirable but pleasant practices, seldom reaches those to whom it is directed and if it does so may have a paradoxical effect. Young men enjoy drinking and getting drunk in concert, and there is an element of rebellion and competition in the drinking style of many young adults: probably the subjects who can take most alcohol and suffer least from hangovers are the most risk-laden for alcohol addiction, but they are unlikely to find that propaganda about the evil effects of drink is in accord with their own pleasant, manly experiences. Temperance propaganda, which unhesitatingly condemns all alcoholic indulgence as evil or damaging, spoils the case by exaggeration. Medical propaganda, relying on the facts of clinical observation, can only point out weakly that 3 or 4 per cent of heavy drinkers will become addicted – too small a proportion to make many young men, confident in their approach to life, change their social patterns.

If legislation and propaganda are impractical for the purposes of preventing alcoholism they may still be useful in causing the alcoholic to present early, before much damage to his intellect, his pocket, his personality, or his health is done. Legislative measures undertaken are many, mostly designed to help alcoholics over immediate crises – which hospitals in general will not and cannot do – at the same time directing the patient's steps towards a treatment centre. In Poland sobering-up stations have been established, where the police take drunks; in the morning the drunk pays for his accommodation and is invited to accept treatment. In the United States various movements, but particularly A.A., have influenced State medical services to provide alcoholic treatment at low rates or free, removing an obstacle to early treatment caused by the very high cost of private practitioners in America.

Propaganda is undertaken on a large scale by many governments: those of Eastern European countries in particular decry the use of hard spirits, while the French Government, though diffident about direct attack and politically unable to reduce quickly the amount of spirits privately distilled, is associated with a campaign designed to moderate the intake of wine. Private organizations, temperance and A.A., are responsible for much of the American propaganda and restriction on liquor advertisements, but State agencies will doubtless take a bigger hand in future.

Facilities for the treatment of alcoholism are being extended rapidly. Since the Second World War, State clinics in the United States have been formed and separate in-patient alcoholic units, relying on group psychotherapy as well as the pharmacological methods of treatment, have been set up. Great Britain, with a small alcohol problem and a great capacity for ignoring what its citizens do in their free time, has lagged behind in the provision of facilities for the treatment of alcoholism, but in 1962 the Ministry of Health invited hospitals to set up small in-patient units for this purpose, asking at the same time for A.A. cooperation in the management of the patients.

The experimental tendency is to set up units separate from the rest of the psychiatric beds, partly in order that group therapy may, by involving a fairly homogeneous segment of patients, be more easily conducted, partly to concentrate experience and developing treatment skill; also, it is felt that alcoholics may jib at entering a psychiatric unit because of the stigma they suppose to attach to such a place. This course is not necessarily the best: group therapy calls for a certain homogeneity, but not necessarily of diagnosis, and groups might operate better if a wide range of psychiatric categories were represented. The treatment of alcoholism as such, while addiction itself remains mysterious, may call for less psychiatric skill than the handling of the patients' auxiliary psychological and social problems, and these require a generally trained psychiatric adviser rather than one specially conversant with the small amount that is known about alcoholism. Research problems are best conducted at a psychiatric centre, where facilities are pooled, rather than at a separate unit at a general hospital without facilities for the run of psychiatric case-work; and the supposition that alcoholics may jib at entering a psychiatric unit because of the shame attached to such a step ignores the widening acceptance of psychiatric services and adds plausibility to the alcoholic's excuses for avoiding treatment – certainly, if an alcoholic is not motivated enough to enter a psychiatric unit he will hardly be motivated enough to cut out alcohol.

The gradual establishment of alcoholic treatment units is allowing systematic research to be undertaken, and from this, whether sociological, psychological, or biochemical, the main improvements of future years must come. It is already clear that there are class distinctions between alcoholics, as between other diagnostic groups of patients: in the United States alcoholism is less prevalent in the skilled artisan group than in the social groups above and below this, while in Great Britain, where becoming an alcoholic costs several thousand pounds, the incidence of alcoholism is highest in the professional and managerial classes – I and II – though alcoholic offences are more frequently committed (or found to be committed) in social class V. The elucidation of the precise social and psychological milieu in which resorting to alcohol is most frequent will be of great interest and, if the social and psychological factors are accessible, practical value; but it is probable that the biochemical basis of addiction itself will, if it is discovered, provide the most striking therapeutic advance.

Chapter 9 started with a description of true drug-addiction – consisting clinically of psychological dependence, tolerance, and the withdrawal syndrome. It is the tolerance – the ability of the altered cell to withstand several (in the case of morphine, more than a hundred) times the standard or therapeutic dose – and the withdrawal syndrome that must have a biochemical basis in altered cellular function.

Descriptively, what happens is that the cell modifies its metabolism and level of activity so as to act virtually normally in the abnormal environment provided by the drug: in the case of alcohol, the cell's method of obtaining energy may also be modified to exploit alcohol rather than, or alongside, glucose. In the absence of the drug to which the cells have become used, their reaction to the prolonged administration of the addicting drug becomes apparent in the withdrawal syndrome, the manifestation of which constitutes the reverse of the actions of the drug – the constipated, relaxed morphine addict with pin-point pupils develops diarrhoea, tension, and dilated pupils; the sleepy, contented, unresponsive drunk becomes, next morning, tremulous, tetchy, and irritable.

This development of tolerance, with its corollary of withdrawal symptoms, is comprehensible as an adaptive mechanism – a biologically useful method of maintaining normal cellular function under abnormal pharmacological circumstances. It is paradoxical, therefore, that the development of addiction should constitute an illness that is usually associated with inadequacy when at a biochemical level it constitutes, if anything, an excess of efficient adaptation. This incongruity is resolved if it is remembered that the inadequate personality (of whatever particular type) is primarily associated with the self-indulgent onset of the illness; the development of addiction in the presence of constant high dosage of the drug, is dependent on other, cellular mechanisms that are not reflected in the patient's personality make-up, and it is these mechanisms that future research must illuminate.

It must by now be apparent that the subject of addiction is one about which much can be said but little is fundamentally understood. The American organization, the Co-operative Commission on the Study of Alcoholism, has the wisest policy that can be made in the circumstances, a statement of which will allow the chapter to end on a realistic note: the Commission is using its funds not primarily for research, but for the organization of a survey of the whole field of alcoholism in order that they may determine where research may most hopefully be undertaken.

Advances in Psychological Testing

There have been many departures from the psychological tests that were in use a generation ago; but most of the work done by scientific psychologists has aimed at establishing basic trends and test-patterns that are associated with general characteristics of the human and animal central nervous systems.

The author has no quarrel with the purpose of this scientific work, but it has not resulted as yet in much data or test-material that is of direct assistance to the psychiatrist. Because of the small practical utility of this work (including, by way of example, the determination of many of the characteristics of the central nervous system as a computer; the elucidation of many of the processes of perception; and an enormous quantity of experimental work on animals) and the fact that scientific psychological testing requires a book to itself, only occasional reference will be made to it and most of this chapter will be concerned with tests that are actually in use in a clinical setting, or are liable soon to become so.

These tests are mostly aimed at making the psychiatrist's subjective judgements about his patients more orderly and consistent and are essentially extensions of his interview: tests such as the Rorschach (ink-blot) test and the Thematic Apperception Test (during which the patient is presented with a series of standard stimuli and is encouraged to display his responses) are not so much additions to psychiatric interviews as substitutes for them.

Over the last few years the Rorschach and T.A.T. tests have been subjected to many experimental assessments and the consensus seems to be that when success is achieved with them this is determined by the skill of the tester rather than the usefulness of the test as such; in other words, the psychologist supposedly diagnosing, say, schizophrenia from Rorschach responses un-wittingly does so from characteristics other than those manifest in the interpretations themselves. The Rorschach, then, the most famous of all the psychological tests, is gradually falling into disuse.

In day-to-day work, psychological tests of a formal kind are little used, and when they are the results are seldom crucial to the diagnosis or management of the case; this statement is as regret-table as it is true. The commonest test employed is the *Intelli-gence Test*; since tests of intelligence first came into use they have been improved and validated against large populations, and ideas about their function have developed considerably. Origi-nally they were intended to determined the *potential* of a subject and the scores achieved were taken to indicate a level that was comparatively fixed and bore little relationship to educational attainment. It is now thought not only that most tests are con-taminated to a considerable degree by questions that can be done best by those taught to understand the lines of thinking that are involved, but that the I.Q. (intelligence quotient) is as much a dynamic measure of current levels of functioning as it is an estimate of built-in capacity. It is therefore no longer a surprise that the I.Q.s of children can increase markedly after a change of environment. Children develop intellectually in a series of fits and starts even under uniform conditions, and this may be exaggerated in the cases of children whose circumstances alter considerably.

Intelligence testing provides us with one of the estimates on which we base a finding of intellectual deficit; in children, this means ascertaining mental defect (or amentia) and in adults, diagnosing dementia. Though very valuable, the test is not all-important, and the management of the defective child, to which ascertainment gives a guide, depends on many other factors, most of them social and in aggregate more important than his test score.

Accurate measurements of the intelligence can be done in adults in whom dementia (loss of intellectual capacity) is sus-pected, but usually the previous level of intelligence can only be roughly estimated from the type of work done, so that precise comparisons cannot be made. On the other hand, in subjects whose dementia has arisen from head-injury and can be expected to remain static, intelligence testing of a sophisticated kind can map out the areas of thought that remain intact and can be exploited in a rehabilitation course.

In certain instances intelligences that lie within the normal range may still be a source of trouble for their possessors. The reader may recall that some patients with objectively normal personalities may find them deficient because of the demands they or their environments make on them – the self-reliant citizen may quail in the commandos and the sanguine senior civil servant become depressed at the denseness of his minister. Similarly the dull but not defective member of a brilliant family may react to his unenviable position by becoming permanently disgruntled or even by making such protests as committing arson, while less frequently but more rewardingly the young person with a behaviour disorder from social class V may turn out to be intellectually superior and consequently out of place. Psychiatrists estimate I.Q.s without tests as general physicians gauge pulse-rates without referring to watches and motorists guess their speed without glancing at the speedometer; occasional checks maintain the accuracy. But of these three endeavours estimation of I.Q. is by far the most difficult, and if the patient is from a different culture or the case presents any anomalies, formal testing is advisable and surprising results are not uncommon.

Otherwise, most psychological tests are as yet insufficiently sensitive and reliable. It is uncommon for psychological test results of a schizophrenic, done before and after effective treatment, to show convincing differences in scores; and even more surprisingly, tests of intellectual function done before and after standard leucotomy may fail to show any difference even though the deficit at interview is gross and unmistakable. It commonly happens that tests which distinguish reliably between two groups of patients (say, a hundred patients before the administration of a drug and the same hundred patients after its ingestion) are not fine enough to be applied with certainty to an individual patient, so that even tests that have obvious advantages and proven applicability in large-scale trials are of no use to the psychiatrist assessing a single person at a time. In the consulting room, for the present, the most searching tests are applied and processed by the interviewing psychiatrist's own central nervous system, still a jump or two ahead of the computers.

The most immediately hopeful practical advance seems to be the drive towards systematizing what the psychiatrist does when he diagnoses and treats his patients. Psychiatrists rely on their interviews because they work, rather than for mystical or jealous reasons, and if parts of the time-consuming assessments could be taken over by psychological tests the new methods would be welcomed.

Some psychological tests are direct developments of interview techniques. A typical example is one used in child psychiatry – the Bene-Anthony test: the attitudes and emotional discords of children are often assessed not by question and answer but by allowing the child to play and noting his preferences for certain obviously identifiable dolls or symbols or activities. The analysis of the child's actions is a skilled task in which, in the many cases where the activity is ambiguous, subjectivity may play an excessively large part. In the Bene-Anthony test the child selects from a large collection a number of figures, each of which he regards as representing a member of his circle, whom he names. He is then given cards to post in slotted boxes attached to each of the figures, and he selects the most appropriate figure when he has read or heard what is written on the card. Since the tests cover a considerable range of attitudes, including antagonistic as well as amicable and dependent feelings, an examination of the cards posted to each of the representative figures can provide a fairly full picture of the child's emotional positions. A test such as this can be administered by non-medical personnel, but the economy thus provided is not its only advantage. By its objectivity it allows the physician who interviews the child's parents and analyses his play to check his own findings and guide him where a conclusion could not firmly be drawn; thus it constitutes a learning device for the child-psychiatrist, improving his performance in his own work.

Refinements of other simple clinical procedures, taking the

form of psychological tests, may allow not only increased skill at the use of the procedure in its clinical form, but the development of theoretical explanations of its usefulness. To take another common example, psychiatric patients are often asked to rephrase proverbs, the form their interpretation takes being particularly helpful in the diagnosis of doubtful schizophrenia. A psychiatrist who uses this test may be able to say that the patient's proverb-interpretation was 'very schizophrenic' but be unable to state quite how the patient's paraphrases differed from those proffered by psychoneurotic or other patients faced with the same task.

In general terms, the acute schizophrenic to whom the psychiatrist says, 'What does it mean when I say "A rolling stone gathers no moss"?' is liable to provide an interpretation that is either concrete ('Well a stone that rolls along couldn't gather any moss, could it? I mean, it's like if a bit of wood or tree rolled along, that wouldn't get mossy either, would it?'), vague and woolly ('A person who – it means a person who, er, it's really nothing to do with stones at all, really. At least. It means if a person does nothing, he won't get very far. No, that's not right.') or simply odd ('If a stone keeps rolling about, you can't pee on it').

Now although odd or strange interpretations may point clearly to schizophrenia, they are not commonly given except by patients in whom the diagnosis is obvious, so that diagnostically they are of little help. Concrete interpretations are given not only by schizophrenic patients but by those who are intellectually dull. Similarly, vague interpretations may be given by patients who do not understand the proverb but do not wish to say so or by those who cannot concentrate on the task. The psychiatrist must therefore regard the interpretations he receives in the light of the total impression gained at interview, and in the absence of a guide to his methods of assessing the interpretations the process remains subjective and difficult to improve, and at the same time cannot be undertaken by less expensively trained personnel.

Recently, objective methods of administering and scoring proverb interpretations have been introduced. These provide a series of problems in which a key proverb is followed by three or four others of which one (perhaps an English version of a corresponding proverb in another language) is equivalent and the others are not. A high score is obtained by patients correctly determining the proverbs that correspond, and the results are easily obtained. But the test, to be used diagnostically, must be taken in conjunction with the results of an intelligence test, since proverb scores are strongly influenced by the patient's intellectual development and allowance must be made for this.

A more economical method of using proverbs in diagnosis has been suggested by the application of psychopathological concepts of the schizophrenic process, briefly mentioned in the chapter on the causation of this illness. The reader may recall that the acute schizophrenic has difficulty in deciding boundaries, and tends to 'over-include': asked to list the names of his family he may go on to list his friends; asked to sort out blocks into groups according to their main characteristics he may sort them not only along the lines of shape and size and colour, but into groups depending on the presence or absence of minute fortuitously formed scratches. These examples of the over-inclusive style of thought may be compared with the vague interpretation of the proverbs. The patient who cannot abstract, who finds himself including all kinds of irrelevant ideas, relapses into formless and unfocused sentences. Correspondingly, the patient who gives a concrete interpretation may do so because he appreciates his difficulty with abstracting the principle and settles for the safe conservative step of simple rephrasing. Even with mundane interpretations, however, the patient displays one characteristic that the woollier patients hold in common – he is prolix: thus those who over-include show this by using a lot of words in their answers, and one objective way of assessing proverb-interpretations for their schizophrenic quality is the simple one of counting the number of words, an observation that may be used in diagnosis without reference to the patient's intelligence quotient.

The psychiatrist makes many observations and provides the patient with a series of fairly standardized stimuli when interviewing. If his techniques of questioning and answer-analysis are scientific, they must contain the germ of an alternative and systematized interview-substitute. Wittenborn and other workers have produced rating-scales that score the patients' behaviour and symptoms, and from which diagnoses can be made. Analysis of this work, which was originally undertaken at least partly with a view to substituting flexible classifications for the rigid and supposedly mutually exclusive diagnostic categories, supports the reality and usefulness of the clinical diagnoses made in previous years but at the same time, by allowing the patient's responses to be scored, provides a way of locating a patient more precisely on the diagnostic map.

Detailed and itemized records of a large number of symptoms and responses, useful though they may be in determining the validity of diagnostic categories in general, are not of much assistance in the management or diagnosis of individual patients at the present time. However, they remain useful research tools. They may be used repetitively on the same patients to follow progress under therapy – though over-frequent use often causes the level of scoring to deteriorate. They may also be used as a guide to outcome or the suitability of different types of treatment; the reader will have noticed that most of the psychiatric treatments, even those called specific, produce cure or effective alleviation in only a certain proportion of the patients treated.

It is reasonable to assume that particular symptoms will provide us with a guide to which treatment to use, if the patterns can be identified. It is already known at a rather coarse level, for example, that the presence of hypochondriacal features makes for somewhat worse results in a depressed patient to whom electric treatment is administered; that a sudden onset makes for a better chance of a remission in schizophrenia; and that evidence of a good previous personality (good meaning conventionally worthy in this instance) makes for a better outlook in almost any psychiatric illness. At a somewhat more subtle level, we know that the depressed patient who shows early waking is rather more likely to respond to the anti-depressive drug imipramine than the patient who does not show this type of sleep pattern but is in other respects similar. But for the most part our ideas about the probable responses of particular patients to agents used in their treatment are based on what we know about the average results of a group of patients so treated; we may have intuitive ideas about whether a patient will do well or not, but these impressions are useless for teaching or scientific purposes. If Wittenborn or other rating-scales are used, however, the results may be retrospectively analysed and the results of therapy compared with the presence, absence, or degree of all the symptoms included on the scale, and pointers to efficient treatment ultimately determined.

Examples of the conversion of simple techniques and tests used at interview into formal, objectively scored tests, sometimes with a theoretical basis over and above their empirical value, could be multiplied tediously, but only one further instance, itself among the most widely used of all, will be given. This is the questionnaire, or inventory type of test. Evidently, the psychiatrist asks many questions which the patient could as easily answer on a form (age, marital status, past history of organic illness, and so on), but many questions more specifically related to attitudes and personality traits could also be posed fairly satisfactorily on a printed sheet.

Questionnaires of one form or another have been widely used in industrial applied psychology: commercial organizations, well aware of the wastefulness of taking on unsuitable personnel, especially in executive positions, and disenchanted with the interview as a means of weighing a candidate's desirability, called on psychological assistance in their efforts to recruit valuable personnel. Commercial psychological questionnaires are usually made up according to the notions of the psychological consultant concerned and are seldom scientifically defensible. Their main disadvantage, however, is not inherent, but dependent on the motives of those who complete them. Few intelligent men fail to spot the questions that need careful answering, and if the post is valuable may be excused for ticking the item that seems most likely to succeed rather than seeking in their hearts for the answer. Some sophisticated questionnaires include items designed to expose liars, but the form of these questions is often suspicious ('I never feel angry at those who beat me when playing games' – tick 'true' or 'false' – or 'I always admit that I am wrong if my arguments are logically demolished') and the candidate who does not identify them does not deserve the job.

The last observation, that the candidate who does not spot the lie question and double up his dishonesty does not deserve the job (i.e. would not do well at it) provides a clue to the rational use of questionnaires: if a large enough series of questionnaires is given to a large enough series of people, and then the later industrial careers of these people are followed up, particular types of scoring pattern can be correlated with particular types of success or failure without regard to the actual phraseology of the questions themselves. Thus it might be found that if 'Yes' were ticked against the item 'I almost always succeed', the employee usually failed, while cool thinking was associated with a tick against 'No' in response to 'I almost always remain calm in emergencies'. Such correlations would not satisfy those in search of honesty, or those judging the questionnaire according to its approximation to objectively determinable facts, but they would be helpful, once the statistical chores were complete, in choosing candidates likely to succeed.

Cattell has followed this pragmatic approach, leaving theory, personal preferences, and unitary tests such as the Rorschach to what he calls 'brass-instrument psychologists'. Essentially, he took all available questionnaires and personality inventories and abstracted from them an enormous list, thousands long, of items. These items were pruned in various ways – by asking trained psychologists to guess what the answer should be and rejecting those easy to see through, by weeding out questions with a threatening content, and so on. A shortened list was then given to a large number of subjects, grouped according to clinical criteria.

Cattell's purpose was to rationalize clinical judgement, and he therefore worked with groups of patients of various diagnostic categories (anxiety-states, hysterical personalities, obsessive – compulsive neuroses, and so on), whose diagnoses had been independently confirmed by several psychiatrists.

Using powerful and complicated statistical techniques, he narrowed his item list further, finally fixing on relatively few questions, all of which showed striking correlations with diagnostic categories or personality traits. For example, in the measurement of neuroticism, he pared his questionnaire down to a forty-item sheet, answerable in ten minutes or so.

Further manipulation of the scores obtained from his mass of subjects enabled him to extract from the results indications that there were several sets of attitudes or response-patterns behind many of the diagnoses even though the diagnoses themselves could be stated in a single word. The neurotic, for example, has four such 'factor-dimensions' in Cattell's formulation, and the forty questions on the appropriate form may be divided up into groups referring to the patient's anxiety, his tendency to pessimism, his degree of dependence, and what Cattell calls his 'tender-minded sensitivity': gross abnormality of two of these sub-test scores would lead to a conclusion that the patient was neurotic, as would mild abnormality in all four, since the scores can be summed.

The questionnaire assessment of the neurotic will be referred to again shortly, but before doing so it is convenient to mention that Cattell has worked not only on neurotic subjects but on the assessment of normal and abnormal personality. His findings differ from those of Eysenck by containing data that require more complicated explanations; for example, Eysenck finds neuroticism to be a unitary factor, with which Cattell, as just described, categorically disagrees.

Unfortunately for psychiatrists, the relative merits of the results of these two workers cannot be compared without a knowledge of the difficult mathematical techniques that are used to process the raw data, and the author, though he finds Cattell's formulations more in accordance with clinical observation than the simple schemata proposed by Eysenck, expects that both sets of ideas will be modified after further work.

To return to the factors making up neuroticism: one of the difficulties about comparing treatments in the neuroses is the near-impossibility of making a fine judgement about the degree of improvement. Still less can improvements of certain aspects of the neuroses be singled out and assessed. However, the use of objectively scored tests enables a satisfactory comparison to be made of the patient's pre- and post-treatment states of mind. Not only may different treatments be compared in this way, but the precise areas of a patient's thinking that are altered might be ascertained. It might be, for example, that only the anxiety and the sensitivity that go to make up neurosis can be altered by psychotherapy, the pessimism and dependence remaining untouched: if this were so, patients could be selected for psychotherapy not according to the degree of their neurosis but for the extent to which their total neuroticism was constituted by the two ameliorable factors; similarly psychotherapy could be directed not against the totality of the condition, with the waste entailed, but against the abnormal factors known to be liable to respond. At present both therapist and patient grope about in the dark. Cattell hopes that, if his methods are used, only the patient need grope, and for a shorter time.

Testing of this kind confirms that the psychotic is different from the neurotic patient and the subject with a personality disorder; the theory that the psychotic was a severe neurotic, or a patient with a personality disorder who responded to the stresses of life with a psychosis instead of a neurosis, does not seem to be still tenable. This kind of testing has also led to the development of objective test-batteries, similar in their mathematical and scientific organization to the questionnaires but depending on test-responses that the patient cannot fake or, in psychiatric work, affect by his desire to produce answers that he feels the psychiatrist may wish to hear.

The impact of this type of work on general psychiatric usage has still to be felt. It has great promise, and though it stemmed from clinical work it has led to the statement of useful and illuminating theoretical ideas, so that it may, in the long as well as the short run, do as much for psychiatric practice as the work of the academic psychologists.

It also contains within it the possibility of extending the availability of psychotherapy. Notwithstanding the criticisms made of psychotherapeutic techniques and results throughout this book, psychotherapy is not only an essential part of the psychiatrist's stock of treatments, but constitutes the most interesting and difficult part of his work. All patients receive psychotherapy of one kind or another, ranging from simple reassurance to prolonged exploratory and re-educational techniques; but since those who need prolonged psychotherapy may be those who are least severely ill or those whose personal assets are considerable, the psychiatrist who does not limit the diagnostic range of his patients may find that after he has completed the essential diagnostic and therapeutic measures on patients who have major psychiatric illnesses there is little time left for pure psychotherapy.

There is no one else to whom the psychiatrist can conscientiously delegate this work, since no other physicians are trained in it and lay practitioners should probably not be allowed to manage patients whose neurosis may turn out, in the long run, to be the consequence of a tumour or an incipient psychosis or a physical illness that sapped the patient's resistance to psychological stress – all requiring medical knowledge for their early diagnosis.

General practitioners see most of the patients in this country who require psychotherapy, and give what help they can. Their prospects of giving more, or more complicated psychotherapy, are restricted by the impossibility of training enough of them adequately and then allowing them the time to practise their skills. To learn psychotherapy, with its few distinct rules and fewer articulate practitioners, a long apprenticeship is needed during which experience programmes the doctor's built-in computer and lays down general rules, not necessarily ones of which he is conscious, for future use. Despite attempts by an enthusiastic group of psychotherapists, headed by M. Balint at the Tavistock Clinic, to tutor experienced general practitioners in the art, it is doubtful whether conventional methods of teaching and practice are adequate ever to allow a sufficiency of skilled practitioners to be available to the patients awaiting treatment.

The development of questionnaires and other tests along the lines proposed by Cattell, despite the mixed greetings given to these supposedly mechanistic methods by the entrenched psychotherapists of the old school, may one day enable assessment and psychotherapy to be simplified to the point where, though sympathy, the gift of concentration, and certain intellectual powers will remain *sine qua non*, treatment may be undertaken by doctors after a much shorter training and with much greater insight and certainty of success.

The practice of child psychiatry, even that which does not concern itself with mental defect, is surprisingly separate from the work done by psychiatrists seeing adult patients. Most of the diagnoses are different and such few as occur in both child and adult sections of the speciality take very different forms. Add to this the consideration that no special predisposition to psychiatric illness in adult life seems consistently to follow psychological disorders in childhood, and that the existence of a history of severe behaviour disorder in early life is the exception rather than the rule with adult patients, and the division between the two disciplines, a real and regrettable one, becomes understandable.

Nevertheless many of the trends in child psychiatry, reflecting the general climate of thought, have been similar to those in adult psychiatry – an inclination to experimental testing of theories, a massive increase in systematic (and inevitably debunking) observation, an exploitation of the latest chemical and pharmocological advances, and a happy development of individual sympathy and respect for the patient with all the liberalization that follows that change.

It may be that now that infants almost always survive to become children, and children to become adults, we may pay more personal attention to them as individuals without risk of pain. When William Gibbon's father called all his five sons William in the hope that one might survive to carry on the family name, he was showing matter-of-fact wisdom, since only one did; his aloofness from all of them until one, the historian of Rome, attained adult life, may have been another form of insurance, no less appropriate to the times. Now that we no longer have to struggle to ensure the survival of the rickety offspring of malnourished mothers but can try to find the best way to order the psychological environment of physically healthy children we wish to know as much as we can about them and the way they react. But we are probably as far from success, as psychiatrists, as the physicians of a century or two ago were in their particular struggle. At this stage in the book the reader will be familiar with the pattern of this sentence: it is not so much that we do not know how people rear their children wrongly (though we do not) as that we do not know how people rear their children. In other words, in the section of psychiatry where theories about abnormality proliferate most luxuriously, we are still largely at the stage of gathering primary data.

However, as always, the maladies themselves have been fairly thoroughly studied, and even after the short term of existence of child psychiatry – almost entirely confined to this century – much may be said about the results of maldevelopment, whatever the mechanisms may be. The study of children divides itself rather sharply into work done on children with intellectual deficit, and work done on the behaviour disorders and illnesses of children who have normal intelligence. Many psychiatrists in the field attend exclusively either one or the other of these two groups (together with such mixed or border-line cases as come their way), a division which must have some practical advantages but is still, like the separation of adult and child psychiatry, a cause for regret.

MENTAL DEFECT (SUBNORMALITY AND SEVERE SUBNORMALITY)

The term 'mental defect' is used here because of its recognizability but commonly today *amentia* is substituted for 'mental defect' and the word *ament* for 'mental defective', in medical practice; administratively the terms 'subnormality' and 'severe subnormality' are now being used. Whatever the choice of term, the meaning conveyed includes the existence of an impaired intelligence, the impairment having been present since birth or an early age, sufficient to make education difficult or, in severe cases, to render leading an independent existence impossible.

Some psychiatrists regard the most mild form of mental defect (feeble-mindedness) as the artefact of our industrialized society with all its intellectual demands, and no doubt it is: however the society exists and in it there is no comfortable place for the illiterate simpleton unless he receives some form of special assistance, so that, since society if it alters at all is likely to do so in the direction of greater complexity, the low-grade variant of normal must be studied and managed and skilfully helped.

A useful distinction is made between the unintelligent person who has no obvious cerebral abnormality and who is usually in the upper range of the subnormal group, and the severely impaired patient, often with obvious stigmata (such as a small head) who is usually at the extreme lower end of the intelligence scale (and would, in the old nomenclature, have been officially classified as an imbecile or, if even more severely affected, an idiot). It is thought that the moderately dull patients are simply variants of normal, the mirror-image in graphic sense of the highly intelligent members of society; they commonly have dull families, as their intelligent opposites have bright families, and it is this group that may be regarded as casualties of social disintegration and technological advance. They are called *subcultural aments*. The 'severely subnormal' patients, on the other hand, usually have some pathological process of a recognizable kind, or are obviously deformed or possessed of multiple handicaps; this group includes such well-known types as the mongols, and the general title give is that of *pathological aments*.

Like other distinctions in psychiatry, that between subcultural and pathological aments is a convenience which, though depending on real differences, takes no account of the many cases that lie on the border-line. It assists clarity of thought and allows some contrasts to be drawn.

The pathological aments have always been known: the 'village idiot', when he was not a schizophrenic, was usually an imbecile, the butt of the local peasants, unable to do productive work at the normal rate. The subcultural aments became a problem when universal education was introduced, though of course degrees of cleverness and simplicity had been recognized before then: they were brought into prominence by the development of intelligence tests, which were originally designed to sort out the children of low potentiality. Like psychopaths, they do not differ from the rest of the populace except in degree and, like psychopaths, they have only lately become and are still only just a medical responsibility, the deciding factor being not the measurable deficit but its social repercussions.

The pathological aments are assumed to suffer from some genetic fault or the consequence of some abnormality in the embryo's intra-uterine environment. The severity of the hazards that the fertilized ovum undergoes is not generally appreciated: about one half fail to develop to term, succumbing at once or after a month or two, often as the result of some disastrous genetic abnormality. Of those foetuses that come to term, one out of twenty has some apparent or latent congenital defect. Of these, a small proportion are pathological aments, and in most cases they are born into families whose intelligence does not differ greatly from the population mean.

These severe aments have been studied intensively; a certain number of them can now be shown to be separate entities, the gross mechanism of the abnormality can be demonstrated in a few, and some can be prevented or cured. Work on a larger scale has pointed the way to general measures of prevention.

The type of pathological amentia for which cure was first found was cretinism. Cretins are short of active thyroid tissue and in consequence develop inadequately; early treatment with thyroid hormone can halt and sometimes reverse the process. Cretins were common in goitrous mountainous districts and the correlation of their incidence with that of women with swollen necks was an ancient observation. These goitres, and cretinism, were associated with a lack of iodine in the food and water of the locality and the routine incorporation of iodine into table salt prevents both goitres and cretinism: cretins are now rarely seen.

A strikingly distinct group of pathological aments are those known as mongols. They received their name from a fancied resemblance to normal members of the Mongolian people when out-dated theoretical ideas about throw-backs and racial inferiority existed. Usually the mongol is an idiot or imbecile, and the condition is not uncommon, comprising about 1 : 1,000 of all births. The *prevalence* of mongolism has risen because of their greater likelihood, now that they need not succumb to the infections to which they are prone, of surviving to middle life and later. In recent years techniques have been developed for examining and identifying the paired chromosomes (the organs in cell nuclei along which the genes are distributed) of animal cells, and the cells of patients with many conditions have been examined to find out if gross chromosomal abnormalities exist. Mongolism is now known to be associated with an aberration of the chromosome conventionally numbered 21, which instead of being paired shows a triple structure (trisomy of the 21st autosome); interestingly, this chromosome is the one found to be abnormal in leukaemic cell studies, and mongols have a greater than average incidence of leukaemia.

Apart from these microscopic studies, which, though of great theoretical importance, do not yet directly assist the practical measures needed to curb the incidence of the condition, detailed studies of the circumstances under which mongolism arises have been done. It has long been known that mongols tended to an even greater degree than most pathological aments to be the offspring of elderly parents: maternal, not paternal, age was the decisive factor, but was not the sole important one that operated. Over a large series it was found that if a mother had had one mongol child the chances of having another depended on her age in an unexpected manner: the older the mother the less likely she was to have a second mongol in subsequent pregnancies; so that the risk of a mother under twenty-five years of age having a second mongol were increased fifty-fold over the average population-risk, while that of a mother over thirty-five was not much greater than the normal risk for the population. This is presumably because, though mongolism is statistically slightly more likely with older mothers in general, its occurrence in younger families means that either husband or wife possesses some permanent chromosomal abnormality that will predispose further conceptions to the production of trisomy 21 and therefore of mongolism. A fairly accurate answer may now be given to the question, spoken or unspoken, about the chances of another mongol birth in a family and the incidence thereby somewhat reduced.

Most pathological aments look odd, and can be ascertained as lacking in intelligence at a glance. Of the ones who do not, one small group, comprising about 2 per cent of the whole, have recently been studied in a brilliantly successful manner. A few aments in institutions, usually fair and active and sometimes with a brother or sister similarly affected, were found to secrete in their urine a particular chemical, phenylpyruvic acid: the condition was described in 1934 and called phenylpyruvic oligophrenia. Its genetic pattern was soon worked out: it is the consequence of the chance junction of two recessive genes, one carried by each parent, which singly produce no pathological results. When two such genes coexist in the fertilized cell the developing infant is unable to deal with a particular and essential constituent of protein food called phenylalanine. The metabolism of this substance is blocked and it is excreted in the urine as an early breakdown product, phenylpyruvic acid: a high concentration of an intermediate substance is the toxic factor that leads to the alteration of a normal newborn infant into a grossly defective child. Phenylalanine, the substance that cannot be completely broken down, is present to harmless excess in normal infant diets; if an infant is secreting phenylpyruvic acid, and the diet is altered so that only the minimum amount of phenylalanine necessary for normal growth and development is given, the toxic breakdown products do not accumulate to a level sufficient to cause cerebral damage, and it is this alteration of diet that has made the condition a preventable one.

In many centres all newborn infants are now routinely tested for phenylpyruvic acid excretion (using the wet nappy) so that treatment may, if it proves necessary, be instituted from the first days, and it is to be hoped and expected that this service will soon become universal. As the child grows and his central nervous system completes its development the dietary supervision can be relaxed but the original metabolic defect, of course, remains unaltered and the adult phenylpyruvic will be a poor risk as a progenitor. Fortunately the carrier – the person without symptoms who possesses a single recessive gene of this type – can now be spotted because of minor alterations in his mode of metabolism of phenylalanine and it may be possible in the future to prevent to a large extent the production of phenylpyruvic infants at all, while those who, having been born since the discovery of dietary treatment, attain normal adulthood will be able to avoid marrying carriers.

Some other uncommon varieties of pathological amentia are also treatable: congenital syphilis responds to anti-syphilitic medication, but because of the low incidence of syphilis itself and the existence of routine checks in antenatal care the condition is now rare. A congenital malformation of the blood vessels associated with a naevus on the face (naevoid amentia, Sturge-Weber syndrome) causes disorganization of one cerebral hemisphere and may, like other conditions (infantile hemiplegia) in which one hemisphere is damaged, be surgically treated in a few cases by total removal of the affected hemisphere, a heroic procedure with a significant mortality. Hydrocephalus, a condition in which the fluid bathing the brain increases in volume and leads to enlargement of the head and attrition of the cerebral tissue, can sometimes be treated by surgical measures designed to allow free drainage of the fluid, often with the aid of tiny artificial valves, but the results are generally disappointing.

For the most part the other forms of pathological amentia cannot be treated in any radical way. This is not to say, however, that they may not be prevented if we know what circumstances are associated with a high incidence of abnormally dull children, and a number of factors of great importance have been determined from recent large-scale studies.

It is very probable that the state of nutrition of the mother during pregnancy is important in some obscure way in determining the incidence of pathological amentia, while there is some evidence from animal work which suggests that the level of nutrition during the period immediately before conception is also of importance. Certainly the relative frequency of pathological amentia has gradually been falling over recent years, during which improvement in nutritional standards has been one of the most notable alterations, while in the concentration camps, where nutrition was pitifully inadequate, the numbers of children born with gross defect was high. Welfare schemes enabling mothers to afford a good and varied diet are therefore of continuing importance, and the optimum level of nutrition is not necessarily that which would be regarded as adequate for the rest of the population, while vitamin supplements, admirable in themselves, are not the answer to the unknown and subtle deficiencies that may lie behind a proportion of abnormal births.

Viral infections of the mother during the first three months of pregnancy may lead to abnormalities, including pathological amentia, in the developing foetus. German measles, in particular, has a deservedly bad reputation for leading to congenital defects – so much so that some obstetricians have been willing to regard an attack of german measles during the critical trimester as an indication for abortion, though only a few per cent of the infected mothers produce malformed or defective infants. General advice can be given to prospective mothers about the childish fevers: if possible, contract them all, and particularly german measles, in childhood; if this is not possible, avoid contacts during the early months of pregnancy.

Most of the congenital abnormalities have a genetic basis: either two carriers of recessive genes contrive to combine two such genes, and produce an abnormal infant (or a non-viable embryo), or a dominant gene forms by mutation and leads to one or other form of defective development. There is a large stock of abnormal genes in the population: probably on average each subject carries four or five recessive genes of potentially deleterious effect, the small number of abnormal children resulting being the consequence of the low chances of meeting a spouse with an overlapping load of abnormal genes and the tendency for such genetically abnormal foetuses as are formed to die *in utero*.

This pool of undesirable genes, both dominant and recessive, is not constant: all arose out of mutations in the first place and fresh mutations occur from time to time, replenishing the stock. Figures from experimental work with small animals such as Drosophila (which is less likely to mutate than man) indicate that radiation is one of the main causes of mutations; furthermore, concrete evidence comes from the follow-ups of pregnant women who were unlucky enough to be near the epicentres of the atomic explosions in Japan in 1945, who gave birth to significantly greater numbers of microcephalic idiots and imbeciles than might have been expected or than occurred in pregnant women farther away from the radiation source. It is quite clear that any increase in radiation leads to a corresponding increase in mutations, the vast majority of which (for practical purposes, all) are harmful. The obvious corollary of such a statement is that procedures entailing increasing radiation should be curtailed. Medically, this is carefully done, X-ray examinations of young women, particularly pregnant women, being reserved for highly necessary occasions.

The nature–nurture argument about intelligence is now outmoded – roughly speaking, genetic factors probably account for rather more than two thirds of observed intelligence, and environmental factors for the rest. Even at its height it was seldom seriously proposed that idiots and imbeciles could have been brought to normal intelligence by improved upbringing. It is interesting, then, that it has been suggested recently that some of the severely subnormal aments are children whose environment has been highly abnormal and adverse. Animal experiments show, as human impressions had made us feel, that organisms bred for intelligence or stupidity, and separated into two contrasting strains, each fairly homogeneous, can be made more intelligent or less so by favourable or unfavourable circumstances. Specifically, dull rats can be made brighter by offering suitably interesting surroundings, while bright rats can be made duller than expectation by the imposition of featureless environments; dull rats cannot be made *duller*, however, or bright rats brighter. Obviously this kind of experiment could not be done on human beings as a planned event. Some unfortunate humans can be observed in dull environments, however, and compared with their peers in better straits: these are the foundling children in orphanages. Results of investigation of these children cannot be relied upon in the same way as animal experiments: for one thing, genetic similarity between the groups compared, far from being approached, is ruled out entirely because the parents of foundling children are often themselves abnormal and dull. It was a striking finding, nevertheless, that infants and young children who were offered the necessities of life as they appeared to the administrators but who were deprived of the intense learning experiences undergone by the normal child as he is fed, clothed, and crooned over, fell far behind in their intellectual development: and there was a feeling, not more, that this lag, once established, could never completely be made up. (This was not the first alarmist story about the psychological ill-effects of institutions for children: those who visited them felt that there must be some ill-effects, so oppressed were they by the thought of having their own children there; some of the better-known theories about *maternal deprivation* have now been shown to be wrong but the disproof of some of the ideas on this topic does not mean that the rest may be shrugged off as scaremongering: the frightful infant mortalities reported early in the century – sometimes almost 100 per cent – were true enough.)

Recently the environments of a group of severe aments without obvious pathology have been compared with those of severe aments of the pathological group, in the expectation that if the environments differed sharply, that of the pathological aments being about normal, those who suspected that environment might play an important part would have their opinions powerfully supported. In the event, support was forthcoming from the facts. Bourne proposes that pathological mothering, the failure to provide the infant with the emotional warmth and attention he craves and relies upon for correct development, lies at the back of many cases of severe amentia. Some factors over and above poor mothering must combine to cause severe defect since many infants who receive little love or guidance grow up without obvious disturbance: probably the severe retardation of motor and verbal skills found in the worst-affected infants and young children is a form of childhood schizophrenia, and does not occur unless the absence of stimulus is combined with constitutional predisposition or, possibly, operates at some critical period. Nevertheless, even if the causation of severe defect by failure of mothering turns out to be a myth or a rarity, the work done has led to an examination of the evidence, which certainly indicates that dreary environment makes the intelligent less so, and prevents the dull from improving. Furthermore, animal experiments (with primates) indicate that it is not enough to provide surroundings which are interesting to explore: before the young of the species will conjure up the courage to pry and examine they confirm that their mother or mother-substitute is hard by.

Without a mother or mother-substitute the young animal remains incurious and the possibilities of the surroundings as educational material are wasted. There are therapeutic lessons, mainly preventive ones, to be drawn from this work. Infants and children need personal and intimate contact and the presence of the mother-figure in order to develop to the full, and there is a chance that the absence of a satisfactory single mother-figure may occasionally lead to a developmental disaster. It follows that infants and young children, particularly those for whom a certain type of life may be ordered such as those who are under the care of the authorities, should be given facilities, emotional and material, that approximate to the organization of the normal family, refined as this is by evolutionary influence.

The large institutions are already gradually breaking up, whether they are for children, adult psychiatric patients, non-psychiatric patients, or prisoners. No large orphanages or homes for children are now being built (except, surprisingly, in New Zealand). The trend, accelerated by talk of dire psychological consequences, is towards fostering the children or, where this cannot be done, the creation of a home-like atmosphere and multiple-family structure within existing institutions. Whatever the rationale for the change, it must be the right thing to do.

Children with cerebral palsy (spastics) have a commoner history of difficult births than most, but it has not been confirmed that the difficult birth itself causes the neurological and intellectual damage. But oxygen-shortage in the foetus and newborn child is probably important and the present tendency is to treat neonatal shock vigorously and to maintain oxygenation at high level.

The Rhesus factor is the start of a sequence of reactions that may occasionally lead to severe deficiency: if the mother's blood does not contain the Rhesus factor and the father's does, the blood of the foetus may contain it. If it does, the mother's blood may develop antibodies against the protein concerned, rather as protective antibodies are developed in the process of resisting an infection. If these antibodies reach a high level and infiltrate the foetus's circulation, the foetal red cells may be affected. In extreme instances the blood of the foetus may be largely destroyed at full term and the baby may be born dead or dying. When the affection is severe the infant is subjected to an exchange transfusion, in the course of which virtually the whole of the blood circulating at birth is replaced by that of a suitable donor. Usually this complication, Rhesus incompatibility, either calls for no treatment or responds well to the measures used, but sometimes an infant survives only to develop slowly and display the characteristic neurological signs of a condition called kernicterus, which is associated with mental defect. These children are casualties, in a sense, of a successful therapeutic procedure, and though the mechanisms are so well understood that the management of rhesus incompatibility is straightforward, it is not easy to see how this type of amentia can be entirely avoided.

The subcultural aments are, as mentioned earlier, our duller but not diseased brethren. Sometimes they find themselves in institutions but since, by I.Q. ratings, the great majority do not, the reasons for compulsory admission to institutions are not primarily those associated with strictly intellectual capacity and are mainly social in nature. They go to institutions because their conduct precipitates administrative action and their I.Q. dockets them in the defective category. In the outside world their poor intellect may be partly responsible for other consequences. They may go to schools for the Educationally Subnormal (E.S.N.), though they are more likely to do so if they are not only dull but troublesome to the teacher of their original class. They may become thieves, prostitutes, or shiftlessly unemployed, though personality factors enter into the selection of these callings more than lack of intelligence, and the contribution of defectives to the crime statistics is often exaggerated. They may develop psychiatric illnesses, particularly because life is more stressful for those who find even simple journeys and calculations effortful occupations, but here again their tendency to do so is smaller than most of the casual estimates imply.

Nevertheless, they constitute a problem as a group simply

because of the way urban twentieth-century society is organized, and it would be helpful if there were some way in which sub-cultural amentia could be reduced. One way, if the results of the animal experiments mentioned earlier may be so transposed, is to improve their education and early upbringing; the latter cannot easily be done, but improved education is having its effect on the recorded I.Q.s of comparable samples of the populace. The main problem, of course, is genetic. In the last analysis, environmental influences are limited by the genetically determined potentiality, and if the subcultural aments are to be reduced in number or degree some way must be found of altering the genetic make-up of the populace.

At the beginning of this century the proposed solution, based on Malthusian logic, was that of eugenics. Part of the reason for setting up the giant institutions for defectives in remote areas and committing to them preferentially those who showed signs of promiscuity was that the country's stock should not be weakened by the offspring of dull and defective subjects. The intellectually superior were enjoined to breed and since the inferior would not restrict their prolificacy there was some agitation for compulsory sterilization (and in some countries statutes were passed allowing this to be done on the grounds of intellectual subnormality). It was noted with alarm that family-size was inversely proportioned to intelligence, and on this basis it was calculated that the average I.Q. in the country would fall a point or two in each generation.

There was a reaction against these forthright views and counsels, which have not been popular for some years. The reaction was mostly emotional, a feature of the humanitarian impulse of the mid century, but such work as was done on the respective I.Q.s of succeeding generations of schoolchildren seemed to belie the nightmares of the Edwardians by showing that the I.Q.s were, even allowing for test-familiarity, rising with the years.

At the risk of lining up with the castrating eugenicists of the turn of the century, with whom I have no sympathy, I feel that the arguments of the anti-eugenicists, now usually accepted on trust, should be re-examined. The arithmetic of the eugenicists, after all, was correct: if large families have low I.Q.s and small families high I.Q.s, on the whole, then the genes associated with the large families will come to occupy a larger and larger share of the genetic pool, and this means, since no one disputes the great importance of genetic factors in intelligence, that a higher and higher proportion of the population will tend to have an I.Q. falling below some arbitrary level such as eighty.

The evidence that I.Q.s are rising in comparable groups of children in succeeding generations is not important to the argument: heights are rising too, by a greater proportion, and both the heights and intelligence scores reflect environmental factors including not only better diet and education but the reduction in serious diseases; the I.Q.s of the girls tested rose more than those of the boys, providing internal evidence that nurture rather than nature was the cause. Improvements in environments and training may thus put off the day when the consequences of genetic dilutions become apparent, but they do nothing about the trend itself. The low intelligence of the pathological aments, as distinct from the subcultural aments, is often the consequence of a single abnormal gene, but that of the merely dull is the consequence of the additive effects of many genes of little individual consequence. Therefore, though advances in genetic knowledge, now proceeding at a great pace as the genetic codes start to crack, may enable us at some time to deal with or prevent the disastrous genetic changes of pathological amentia, it is highly unlikely that within the foreseeable future the multiple genes concerned in subcultural amentia will become amenable to intervention.

This brings us to the nub. There is only one other way of controlling the genetic make-up of the people as a whole, and that is by eugenics. Negative eugenics, meaning the prevention of breeding by the poorly endowed, is not a popular or entertainable proposition; certain countries undertake sterilization or castration of a compulsory kind, thinly disguised as voluntary by getting the patient to have it done in order that his request for freedom may be more favourably considered, but usually the grounds are mainly those of some type of criminality. Legislation of this kind could never be introduced in the United

Kingdom. Positive eugenics, meaning the encouragement of large families in the intelligent groups, has more to be said for it.

Another method, at present of minor importance, has some influence on the genetic pool – that of artificial insemination. In the future social changes may make it easier for the childless woman to have a family, and the consistent use of donors of moderately higher intelligence than the mother would constitute positive eugenics of a sort; donors of excessively high intelligence, though it is tempting to indulge in fantasies about their effects, might make for emotional discord between the resulting children and their mothers.

Having discussed the possible curative measures and found them to be few, and considered the preventive measures and found them to be largely impracticable, it remains to mention what can actually be done for these patients.

The earliest steps that can be taken with pathological aments are those designed to assist the parents of the afflicted children. Even in the recent past it has happened all too often that the parents have received inadequate information. Occasionally the abnormality has first been pointed out to the parents not by a doctor or nurse, but by a neighbour, and parents' comments on this failure on the part of their medical advisers have been understandably bitter. Though the details of the transaction will vary with individual families, it is often best to tell the father first, soon after the infant has been ascertained to be defective, and either to tell the mother later or, if he desires it, to let the husband transmit the information.

There are then questions that should be answered at once, and repeated later; these questions may not always be explicitly put by the parents but it is the doctor's duty to abide not by the rules of evidence but by those requiring him to assist his patients as best he can. Parents will want to know whether it is necessary or advisable for the child to go to an institution: no hard and fast answer can be given, but it is probably best for the child if his early years are passed with the family, since no institutional training can compete in intensity with that provided by a mother, though later on his training may be more effectively completed in an institutional setting. Often they will wish to have another child, sometimes for self-reassurance, and they should be told the odds of recurrence if these can be judged; the mother who decides to keep a severely affected child at home may wish to avoid further conceptions and should be offered the contraceptive advice which women so frequently hesitate to ask for. The parents should be told of the course that development will take, covering the time from infancy to adulthood.

The permanent nature of the disability should be firmly stated. The hidden expenses of keeping a severely defective child at home should be deduced from the duties that this will involve, duties that prevent the mother from going out to work. The doctor should make it known to the mother that there are agencies that can assist and advise her without prying, put her in touch with the National Assistance Board if her circumstances are hard (whether or not her husband is working), and try to assist her to obtain preferential housing if the present accommodation is poorly provided with sanitary equipment or reasonably sound-proofed walls.

There is no disguising the fact that the path of the mother who keeps a severely subnormal child at home is a hard one, but the decision about the future of the child should be left with the family and this may conscientiously be done – if they are in possession of enough data to make a judicious decision. Some institutions will now agree to accept children for a month or so at a time once a year to give mothers who are looking after them a rest, or a chance to take a holiday with the rest of the family; the effect of the defective child on his brothers and sisters seems to be small and need not be considered seriously in making plans for his early years.

The central method used in the management of aments, both the pathological aments who have just been considered and those subcultural aments whose disability makes ordinary schooling unsuitable, is training. In early years training in cleanliness and social graces is needed, and must continue for longer than with the average child, since the defective not only matures more slowly but takes longer to come to the end of his intellectual development. It used to be the intention, after the first few years, to train the growing child to do some kind of handicraft or trade, and the things the child was given to do resembled those given to adult patients by the older generation of occupational therapists. Certain changes have taken place that make this course no longer the best, though it remains a pleasant and interesting one for the patient: the older trades are now almost extinct; the tendency is to try to get the patients out of the institution altogether if possible, and if not, then to get them out to work. Therefore patients are now trained in order to fit them for unskilled or semi-skilled employment. To work with normal colleagues the patients need to be pre-trained over a long period, taught the value of money and the way it can be better earned by greater output, and taught to read and write simple words. If the patient has no gross defect of personality he may be able to compete very successfully with workmen whose intelligence is average for their group; and at some tasks, notably the most boring and repetitive ones that modern industry has to offer, he may beat them.

At present, with virtually full employment, these patients often become fully independent citizens. If the economy fails to maintain the present level of employment, community care of defectives may run up against difficulties, in common with that of psychotic patients, though the latter, being rather slow, may become casualties of an increase in unemployment before their duller brothers. In the future, furthermore, the most automatic and simple tasks in industry are likely to be automated – it is surprising to an outsider that so many repetitive tasks still remain. When the effects of automation are felt to the full the employment of subnormal patients and the upper reaches of the severely subnormal group will become harder to arrange. There remains one segment of industry, the largest, that is still principally run by hand – the massive effort of preparing food and doing housework undertaken by the housewives of the country in their own homes. If the stigma the rich laid on 'service' can be removed before automation is fully achieved, help in the home and the garden, with all the rationalization of effort that this implies for those mothers who can be employed more valuably and enjoyably at other skilled tasks, may come to the assistance of the defective who is trained and willing and wishes, like any-one else, to lead an independent life.

FUNCTIONAL DISORDERS IN THE YOUNG

Children suffer not only the functional illnesses seen among adults but a variety of others, loosely known as behaviour dis-orders, many of which are the protests they make against the hardships that beset them.

Schizophrenia in childhood has already been described (Chap. 1), and is probably a variant of the adult form. Though the clinical appearance of the childish schizophrenic resembles that seen in adult practice only approximately, some of the psychopathological aspects and the genetic pattern are very similar. Recurrent depressions are rarely seen in childhood, and usually take some atypical form such as generalized nervousness (a few cases of school-phobia may have a depressive basis); in retrospect it is sometimes possible to recognize depressive episodes in the childhoods of those who suffer frequent depres-sions in adult life, but children have labile moods and it is seldom that the depressed state is recognized as psychotic at the time.

Children may also suffer the dementing consequences of head injury or encephalitis, and if they are unfortunate enough to be affected in this way develop slowly and uncertainly like those brain-damaged from birth; sometimes, especially after ence-phalitis or in the presence of certain types of epilepsy, they show a special inclination to antisocial behaviour. Their psychoneu-roses are usually evanescent and of obvious origin, with a better outlook than the illnesses seen in adults. Though they do not suffer, with very rare exceptions, the degenerative diseases of late adult life, they have another set of conditions to sustain in their place.

These states, the *behaviour disorders*, are for the most part similar in their quality to activity seen in children in general, but cause concern because they occur in an exaggerated form or because a normal phase is unduly prolonged. There has been a tendency, now corrected, to equate behaviour disorders with naughtiness or unsightliness or other adult criteria of abnormality. Thus many papers have been written on thumb-sucking, nail-biting, masturbation, and negativism as if these were pathological. There seems to be a general acceptance of the new proposition that these activities are essentially normal and do not need treatment. Placid children suck their thumbs, seem to enjoy it and do no harm. Active children bite their nails, seem to enjoy it and do no harm. Curious children learn how to masturbate and make no bones about enjoying it; and parents are now usually able to accept that it does not blind or derange its *habitués*, if only from their own experience.

Negativism – the tendency to favour the word No and do the opposite of what is suggested – may need tactful handling but constitutes a passing and universal phase; in adult terms it is a form of naughtiness, now also recognized by astute psychiatrists to be rather common. Food refusal is a syndrome that is confined to subcultures where there is no food shortage; it may usually be taken to mean that the highly artificial feeding patterns of adult society are being forced on the child and is almost invariably associated with a normally increasing weight; mealtimes provide the child with rare opportunities for revenging himself on adults and, if his contrariness seems excessive even when tensions and watchfulness that have arisen secondarily are allowed for, the background of the dilemma should be explored before the parents are told to refuse to enter into emotionality at table and the child is thereby robbed of his weapon.

Even if parents complain of only the most mildly troublesome activity undertaken by their child, activity that is well within normal limits, the fact that the parents have thought it, or the unease that underlies it, sufficiently worrying to make them go to the trouble of arranging a consultation indicates that the matter calls for more than simple reassurance on the score initially cited. Some other behaviour disorders are uncommon enough to indicate, *a priori* of themselves, that unusual factors must be operating and require closer investigation. Grossly excessive waywardness may indicate a specific disease process, or may be associated with irrational or uneven (rather than loving or punitive) discipline; temper-tantrums may reflect a violent unrestrained family atmosphere; tics, friction between one or other parent and the child (often compounded by the parent's irritation at the habit itself); abandonment of previously established toilet-training, aggression called forth by some aspect of the current life-situation. These vignettes of causative factors show that, despite our recent acceptance of the individuality and dignity of the child patient, he is not truly an independent being; he is the creature of those who surround him and at the mercy of the stimuli they impose.

It is apparent that any reliable statements about what may be accepted as normal and what merits treatment of some kind must depend on the existence of a body of objective data about the upbringing of children and their reactions to the strains imposed. With so many childish upsets representing variations on a normal central theme, this data is more important as an aid to the treatment of children than it is with adults because of the preponderance, in adult work, of marked and unmistakable deviations from normal conduct or thinking. Child psychiatry is still far from ideally equipped with this background knowledge but, for a speciality that hardly existed before the beginning of this century, the quantity already ascertained is imposing and the schemes under way well-planned and extensive.

The soppier ideas about innocent children could hardly survive Freud's onslaught, but though we may admire his verve and self-confidence the fact remains that he wrote a book on child psychology years before he saw a child as a patient. Some modification of his original ideas has inevitably taken place as first-hand observations have been added to the accounts his hysterical patients gave of their early years. The emotional development of children has been followed at an individual level by the post-Freudian psychiatrists, and apart from the particular theories that have been proposed, methods of communication with the child have been remarkably improved. The analysis of the child's play, in particular, has enabled the limitations of the small and conventional vocabulary of the young, wary child to be circumvented. As in other psychoanalytically oriented studies, the work has been mainly a refinement and elaboration of the original theses, with a preponderance of attention to the sexual and emotional rather than the intellectual development of the child.

Work on young animals has thrown interesting light on the possible significance of stages in the mental growth of humans. In particular, the description of sensitive periods in the young animal's early days, during which critical relationships such as a positive attachment to the mother-figure are automatically established but before or after which such relationships form slowly or uncertainly, provide a way of explaining the different reactions of children of different ages to identical stimuli or deprivations. Animal work also shows some evidence that the prevention of basic activities, such as sucking, makes for a long-term tendency for the animal to suck later in life (and it has been suggested that smoking may be in part a consequence of restricted childhood sucking), though the existence of unitary or binary drives (Freudian sexual drive or in the antithetic formulation of later years *eros* and *thanatos*) is not confirmed. Jean Piaget has complemented Freud's work on the personal emotional development of the child by examining the manner in which the intellect expands; his descriptions of the balance struck between the twin processes of developing intellectual models of the outer world in the mind, and the modification of these models by reference to reality are illuminating; imbalance (with too many uncorroborated models and schemata) smacks of withdrawal, and the reverse (with too little orderly assimilation), of inconsequential imitativeness, both of these being states seen in everyday practice.

Rather like the most reliable work on old people, mentioned in the following chapter, surveys of childhood development are best done by following a cohort of children from birth to late adult life. The child patient is, it goes without saying, important in his own right, but much of the potential value of child psychiatry lies in the hope (rather than the expectation, it now seems) that the modification of early influences will materially reduce the incidence of the severe illnesses of adult life; even a demonstration of environmental or social factors associated with the milder upsets of adolescence or early adult life would be of great assistance. These studies, necessarily very time-consuming, were started even before the Second World War in the United States and are being pursued now in Europe. The children selected for study constitute a normal population and there is no hope of obtaining, from the two or three hundred children that any one group of researchers can follow, more than a sprinkling of children who are significantly psychologically disturbed. Therefore, though a single survey of this type would give useful information about patterns of upbringing, it would not produce reliable and reduplicated evidence about causative factors in the illnesses of the children who became psychiatric casualties either as children or in adult life. In order to circumvent this disadvantage the several European longitudinal surveys have been coordinated so that the basic methods and criteria are interchangeable, and within a few years large amounts of compatible data should be available for examination and analysis. It is worth remarking here that the comparative normality of the children who are brought to child psychiatry clinics means that one of the most useful tasks that these clinics can perform is the detailed examination of normal upbringing. Even if no more could be determined than a means of dividing childhood anxieties into those necessary as learning experiences and those better avoided, a great humanitarian advance would have been made.

Even apart from these orchestrated studies, the most casual surveys undertaken constantly show that things are not what they seem. Well-known articles have been written about the probable linkage between an allegedly rising incidence of peptic ulceration and the imposition by modern mothers of strict time-table feeding and early weaning, when in fact demand feeding and late weaning turn out, on inquiry, to be the prevalent mode. The most flagrant over-generalizations have been concerned with the particular behaviour disorder known as delinquency, a topic that merits separate consideration.

JUVENILE DELINQUENCY

Delinquent acts correspond to behaviour disturbances seen in clinical work except that for delinquents the authority affronted by the conduct is organized society rather than the parent. None of the more obvious and facile explanations of delinquent behaviour holds water, as Barbara Wootton showed incisively in *Social Science and Social Pathology*. Delinquency is apparently on the increase, though no one can really tell: more official attention is almost certainly paid to misconduct today than it was, say, when Stalky shot cats with his pistol and tortured, terrorized and trespassed his way through adolescence. It is certainly a normal phenomenon, in the same sense that it is very common. Many who speak indignantly of the larcenies committed by boys in increasing numbers (up to the age of fourteen) forget their own light-fingered escapades or, if they remember or are reminded of them, dismiss them as frivolous or trifling. Many who deplore the hooliganism of the late teens forget or dismiss their own rioting on Boat Race Night or after the Lord Mayor's Show, Guy Fawkes processions or an important rugger match. Nevertheless, there is a widespread feeling that, though the statistics may be ludicrously unreliable, the real incidence of juvenile delinquency is on the increase, and on occasion psychiatrists are called upon to offer advice.

Like its major variant, adult crime, juvenile delinquency is not strictly a medical affair. As with crime, the more serious the delinquency, the higher the proportion of personally disturbed subjects involved: but even the most serious delinquent acts are done by lads of whom the majority are, apart from the evidence provided by the acts themselves, normal.

Research on delinquency has been done in much the same way as that on the behaviour disorders of childhood. Most of the studies inquiring into particular antecedents of delinquency have been, when uncontrolled, misleading and, when controlled, inconclusive; not all the preceding circumstances can be ascertained and inquiry is focused according to the inspiration of the researcher so that the well-conducted work done has provided an unusually large negative literature: delinquency is *not* due to broken homes, inadequate clubs, intellectual dullness, revolutionary upheaval, and so on.

Nevertheless, some positive findings accrue. Delinquents who are caught are *on average* on the dull side of normal, are usually said (except by the Gluecks) to be less robust or to have more adverse physical factors than the average, commonly come from poorer than richer families (again, except in the United States, where social class and delinquency do not relate), learn something from delinquent subcultures operating after the age of seven, and may have been laxly disciplined by parents who cared neither for each other nor their children. These findings are far too imprecise for predicting whether delinquency will or will not take place in a given child. As with adult crime, easily the best guide to a future career of delinquency is not the psychology of the individual but the state of his record.

The Gluecks, in the United States, have made heroic efforts to work out factors that could be incorporated in a formula serving the ends of the prediction of delinquent patterns in non-delinquent children; recently similar work has been started here. As with studies of psychiatric conditions, the ideal method is a longitudinal one, with a normal group of unselected children, taken as the starting-point of the study and followed for many years.

TREATMENT

Child-guidance or child-psychiatry clinics are increasing in numbers at a rate that is high even in such a mushrooming speciality. Much of the early interest in children was concerned with educational failure, and about one third of the country's clinics are run by the Ministry of Education, which has a share, with the Ministry of Health, in the management of another third. This division is unsatisfactory, but its end will depend on whether the majority of the conditions seen in children turn out to be suitably managed by whatever methods psychiatrists are, by then, using, or to be largely matters of re-education in the didactic sense. About four children in every thousand attend these clinics.

If any treatment is given it is usually psychotherapeutic in nature: the physical, pharmacological, and administrative advances in adult psychiatry have not proved to be transferable to work with children. Psychotherapy is applicable more to the parents than the child, but if the parents are abnormal they may not be persuaded to cooperate, while even if they are quite willing to assist they may not be able to attend the regular daytime sessions that are desirable. Because therapy is, perforce, child-centred, the psychoanalytical techniques and interpretations, which focus on the individual, are widely used in this type of psychotherapy.

The results of treatment are hard to ascertain. Follow-up studies designed to show the long-term effect of therapy on disturbed children are few, and those invoking controls purport to show that the giving or withholding of treatment makes no difference at all in the long run. Whether this is so or not, the treatment still probably lessens the child's distress at the time, providing him with an uncritical ally in an unfriendly world. Uncontrolled work, offering no comparisons except with a mental image of what might have happened had the treatment not been given, are manifestly unreliable; the more so since it is becoming apparent that anxiety states and obsessive-compulsive conditions of moderate severity or worse (by adult measure) may be found in more than a third of randomly selected children at any one time, the corollary of such a finding being that the untreated prognosis must be excellent and that the existence of these fear and insecurity states must be part of normal childhood.

Compared with adult psychiatry the practice of child psychiatry, despite its rapid expansion and wide acceptance, is in the doldrums. Child psychiatrists have to accept that much of the knowledge gained in adult work is useless in their own field, but the critical approach fostered among workers with adults has not found corresponding favour with them. The application of scientific principles to the practice and assessment of psychotherapy is always beset with great difficulty, and the nature of medical treatment makes it impossible to conduct a formal prospective controlled trial of the most informative type; also the good outlook in many of the disorders means that superficially there is no urgency about the elimination of the less effective treatment methods. But in a branch of the speciality that carries so many hopes of eliminating adult maladaptations and occupies so many workers, both medical and ancillary, it is obviously necessary that they should brush vested interests aside and examine more closely the variety of treatment methods that are hopefully and intuitively applied.

13   Old Age

There has been a considerable and world-wide increase in the psychiatric illnesses associated with old age during the last generation or so. Reasons for the absolute increase in the numbers of old patients presenting to psychatrists are easy enough to discern; over the last half-century the life-span in Russia has approximately doubled, and even in countries where less primitive initial conditions obtained the expectation of life has increased from fifty or so years to something approaching seventy.

This change in longevity was due, at one time, mainly to public health measures and improved nutrition; later the specific anti-bacterial agents added to the effects of large-scale preventive work. The most obvious tendency was for these preventive and curative measures to allow more people to reach middle age, rather than greatly to increase the life-expectation of those middle-aged subjects who had struggled through the hazards of youth; such diminution in fatal infectious illnesses as has taken place for the middle-aged seems to have been almost balanced by an increased incidence of other fatal conditions, including particularly coronary artery disease: thus the number surviving to the late sixties and early seventies is more markedly increased than the number attaining great ages of seventy-five and over. It follows that we should expect that a rise in the numbers of psychiatric illnesses associated with old age, corresponding in magnitude to the increase in the population would be found. It is an interesting and rather sombre observation that the amount of illness seen is much greater than the rise in numbers of the aged could possibly account for.

Various explanations of this disturbing finding are heard from time to time. The most popular is that families are not what they used to be, that the young people have not the same sense of responsibility as once prevailed, and that many aged are simply cast adrift. Some evidence of a coarse type, such as that implicit in a lower incidence of senile psychosis in rural compared with urban districts, seems to point to social factors, but the informed consensus is that the younger generations accept their responsibilities in an admirable fashion. The suggestion that the aged have always shown signs of mental disorder, but have only lately had the opportunity of obtaining treatment, is more likely to account for a part of the higher incidence; but the psychoses of old age, unlike the neuroses or personality problems of the young, are not episodes that can be shrugged off or hidden, at a pinch, from associates. With the exception of mild depressions, most of the psychoses of old age force themselves on the attention of others and could not have escaped notice even before the spread of psychiatric services. No new pathological processes beset the brains of today, so far as is known, and indeed the adverse effects of alcohol and syphilis are less commonly seen; it is possible that certain patients suffer in later life from the consequences, not noted at the time, of a poor supply of oxygen to the brain during anaesthesia, exposure to low concentrations of carbon monoxide, or the effects of mild head injuries, but these hazards could hardly account for more than a fraction of the increase recorded. One possible explanation, of an unhelpful but comprehensible kind, is that those who now survive and who would formerly have succumbed, are mentally less durable as they are biologically less naturally viable; perhaps, as some workers have said, those who formerly survived to a great age constituted, on other grounds as well as their longevity, a biological and intellectual *élite*. It is in accordance with this formulation that the intelligent are found to weather the years better, retaining flexibility long after their duller contemporaries; and that the incidence of organic mental illness, like that of several other major illnesses, is strikingly greater among the lower than the upper social classes. Another explanation, also unconfirmed but of some importance if true, is that some change is taking place in the nature of ageing, the effect of which is malign.

Old age carries with it a greater risk of serious psychiatric illness than does any other epoch, and together these illnesses constitute the greatest cause of disablement at the close of life. With the different methods and policies for younger patients altering the picture in mental hospitals, dementia is now becoming the commonest cause of a stay of more than two years, and of the aged patients admitted for organic degenerative disease of the central nervous system, probably less than ten per cent are discharged. If present trends of disease continue, intellectual decline is likely to become the most common of all the causes of admission to hospital.

NORMAL AGEING

The psychoses of old age differ from the changes seen in what may be called normal ageing and are not simply a caricature of these. The evolution of the youth, hot for certainty and reform, into the complacent and conservative old man, has been chronicled by many able pens and is part of our common experience. Familiarity should not blind us to the unreliability of much of our data on normal ageing, however. The scientific work done has been largely *cross-sectional*, which is to say that old people have been compared with middle-aged and young people living at the same time. Though the most obvious differences between the generations can be disclosed by this type of comparison, the results are on the whole over-pessimistic about the older groups. *Longitudinal studies* follow a cohort of subjects from youth to old age, comparing the same group at different stages in their lives, and throw a rather different light on the process of growing old, showing, for example, that intelligence, at least in those of high intelligence, increases for much longer than had been supposed – until as late as fifty years; and that liberality of thought and outlook increases until middle years, the apparently early onset of reactionary patterns noted in cross-sectional studies being a consequence of failure to allow for the effects of an increasingly liberal culture.

Even if our facts and figures about the psychology of the aged are still uncertain, clinical description of the changes brought about by normal ageing is full enough for our needs. Usually the old person is less immediately able to remember recent events than once he was, becomes more orderly or pernickety, loses some of his capacity to feel deeply, and slows up at certain types of task; some of his altered activities, such as the slowing, are the direct consequence of ageing changes, while others, such as the orderliness, represent his attempts to adjust to his altered capacity. Still others are the comprehensible psychological reactions of subjects who find their prestige, income, power, and ambitions waning inexorably as they gradually join one of the oppressed minorities of the country.

Psychiatrists, at the present stage of medical care, are mainly concerned with the severe illnesses of the aged, in which social factors, though important, do not commonly play a principal part. It would not be out of place to comment on what will no doubt become relatively more important as the more dramatic events of the later years of life become better controlled – the poor social circumstances of many of the aged in our midst. Because of the general acceptance of the age of sixty-five as a suitable one for retirement many fully employable people are idle; the advisability of continuing work after a certain age depends not only on the individual but on the work involved. Where experience is at a premium, prolongation of the working life is desirable, though it may not be if speed or agility is needed.

The fact that a decision about whether an employee should retire or not may be embarrassing is not a sound reason for adhering to an arbitrary, and by now outdated, age-limit. Many old people do work at new jobs after formal retirement, despite the financial discouragements and many who do not, do not want to; but a large number exist in wasteful and enforced inactivity, on the pittance provided by the State, as a consequence of entirely mutable administrative rules. Some of these old retired men and women live alone, some are house-bound, and many more find difficulty in walking. Yet very few are visited by any representative of a welfare organization and, what is more to the point, since visits are not necessarily welcome, many do not know what services are available to them. There is obviously much to be done to try to provide a fuller life for the older generation.

GENERAL MEDICAL FACILITIES

Medically too, this is a depressed area. The old patient is not easy to get into hospital because of the fear that the bed will become 'blocked' by a chronic case; and though old people do almost as well as young in terms of return of function after a spell in a general ward, the scarcity of long-stay geriatric beds for the chronically ill does mean that patients are sometimes admitted to an acute unit at the request of general practitioners when chronic care is obviously necessary.

The deficiency in the numbers of long-stay beds for old people is alarming, and the effects pervasive. No acute geriatric unit can run efficiently unless it is backed by long-stay beds where patients who fail to respond completely can be transferred, and any acute unit without such support soon becomes full of long-stay patients, with all the wastage of special investigational equipment and staff that this entails. Yet capital expenditure in this growing field is relatively less than in most others; it should be more, to make up the large gap, and more still because the gap is growing.

Some of the repercussions of geriatric deficiencies are felt in the mental hospitals. Old, sick, lonely people are usually sad enough to qualify for admission to such a hospital if they and their family doctor can think of no alternative, and the large psychiatric hospitals can always fit another chronically ill person in. Many of these patients should not be in hospital at all, and are admitted mainly for social reasons. Still more of them are not psychiatric patients in the proper sense of the term, and should not be in psychiatric hospitals; so long as there is nowhere else for them to go they are, of course, welcome, but though their numbers are small they take up a disproportionate amount of the time of psychiatric nurses whose training fits them better for other tasks. To some extent, then, the difficulties in the psychiatric hospitals are the indirect consequences of the wide gaps in social and medical geriatric services throughout the country.

THE PSYCHOSES OF OLD AGE

It is only in the last generation that the separation of the different illnesses of this stage of life has been done with any accuracy. Many of the illnesses are attended by a rapid deterioration, and the poor prognosis of the group of patients as a whole must have caused much of the lack of interest in geriatric psychiatry that existed. Also, to the superficial observer, there is little difference between the clinical pictures presented by representatives of the diagnostic groups; all are old, many are inert, or querulous, or paranoid, or confused, or neglected. Nevertheless, there are clear-cut distinctions to be drawn between different categories of illness, distinctions that allow effective treatment to be used in many cases.

The first group of illnesses that may be distinguished is the functional psychoses – affective illnesses (mainly depressions), and schizophrenia. These occur fairly frequently and take forms that, if the psychological and cultural influences of age are allowed for, do not differ notably from corresponding illnesses seen in the prime of life. Recognition that the inert, expressionless, unkempt patient with ideas relating to death and unworthiness, perhaps with some old-fashioned topic like masturbation for mumbled self-reproach, could be returned to normal with electrical treatment, and that the suspicious, hallucinated querulant without intellectual deficit or loss of the power of logical thought could be tranquillized to the point of social acceptability and personal ease of mind has done much to reduce the misery of old age.

Another group of patients enters hospital in a delirious state. For some, this is simply an episode in the course of a progressive dementia and the treatment that is given is only palliative. But for others, chiefly identified by the absence of any other indication of mental deterioration, the delirium constitutes an illness in its own right, for which the cause may never be found but from which recovery, if it takes place, is likely to be complete. Investigation and treatment of these delirious patients is a matter of some urgency, since the episodes carry a mortality of nearly 50 per cent.

With uncommon exceptions, all the other aged psychiatric patients enter hospital with illnesses that have as their principal feature loss of intellectual capacity – the dementias. Certain subcategories of dementia constitute recognizable disease entities, others are secondary to tumours or disease elsewhere in the body, and a few are treatable. For the most part all that is to be found is a degeneration of the intellect and the personality, with nonspecific pathological findings, having as their main common feature a reduction in cerebral mass. For the most part, it would be easy to add, the problem is one of ageing rather than disease.

This antithesis is only tenable if ageing is regarded as something inevitable and normal, separate from disease. There is no reason to suppose that this is the case. Ageing changes are not universal among animals, and they vary widely among men. Research into ageing processes is the most important aspect of geriatric medicine though the social disruption that will follow any major advance can hardly be imagined.

Ageing, whatever it is, has something to do with mutations or mutability. It is associated with an increased liability to develop most cancers, and a decreased liability to develop others. It may be speeded up by radiation. In a certain rare illness it may develop at galloping speed. It is also a characteristic that provides species-benefit in our culture, if followed quickly by death, since it rids the offspring of the need to support a parent or provides the offspring with a share of the amassed goods of the parent, enabling a larger complement of children (carrying corresponding ageing genes) to be reared. Thus ageing changes, or diseases of old age, may be said to propagate themselves by processes allied to natural selection, and it is reasonable to expect that they will increase gradually. It is to be hoped that research into mechanisms by which the diseases exert their effects will prevent the manifestation of the predisposition, but at present there is no indication that research into the most prominent pathological processes is on the point of producing results.

PSYCHIATRIC FACILITIES

Some patients live with their families, though in advanced

senile illness the patient can only be managed at home if the house is virtually converted to a hospital. Some are to be found in accommodation for the aged sick, principally old workhouse buildings. The majority live in the geriatric wards of large psychiatric hospitals. For those suffering from functional psychoses and delirious states the psychiatric hospital is suitable enough; as suitable, at all events, as it is for psychiatric patients in general. Different accommodation is needed for those who will need to stay indefinitely and for patients whose deficits are social rather than medical. Whether new and centrally sited accommodation will be forthcoming under Ministerial plans for hospital development (reviewed in Chapter 6) remains to be seen. The old people suffer from having no one to speak up for them and a short voting life left, but the facilities provided for them at present seem worse than even these grave deficiencies warrant.

The Impact of
Psychiatry on the Law

Psychiatry and the law are ill-suited but their uneasy marriage persists through sheer necessity. From time to time psychiatrists enter courts to give expert evidence, often losing face in the process, while occasionally lawyers draft some new statute covering the acts of the psychologically ill, usually in such a way as to flout what psychiatric knowledge is available. Lately, both psychiatrists and lawyers have been doing rather better.

The subject of *psychiatric testimony* is one that has emotional associations for all concerned. Like other doctors, psychiatrists feel duty-bound to testify on matters of fact, whether or not they approve of the litigation that is going on; even if they refused they could always be served with a subpoena. In general psychiatrists also feel bound, if asked, to give expert testimony, meaning the interpretation of facts for a jury. But few enjoy testifying and for most the whole process is tiresome and disturbing.

At one time psychiatrists were seldom called in criminal cases, except for capital charges or to bolster the exposition of extenuating circumstances. Of late the spread of awareness of the importance of mental states in determining culpability, together with recent statutes reflecting this, have made for an increased demand for psychiatric testimony. Civil cases have always included their share of points of psychiatric interest, with disputes over grounds for divorce, testamentary capacity, and so on.

If a man is charged with a serious offence, particularly murder, the prosecution frequently obtains reports on his mental state. If he seems sane or is at any rate not clearly insane, the trial proceeds. The defence may decide, if the patient is odd or the case impossible to defend in any other way, that the prisoner's mental state will be exploited to reduce the penalty. In the case of capital murder, where any alternative is preferable to the death-penalty, the defence of insanity or some lesser psychological abnormality is frequently raised. The defence solicitors solicit psychiatrists of medico-legal or local reputation to examine the prisoner with a view to giving them a report on him. If the report is in accordance with the story they wish to present to the jury, they arrange for him to give evidence. If it is not, they ask another psychiatrist. In this way the prisoner is reasonably assured that someone will be found, at the sixth or seventh attempt if necessary, to say that he is not absolutely normal.

The prosecution may counter by obtaining the services of psychiatrists who, having examined the prisoner, believe him to be normal enough. By the time the case comes to court there are psychiatrists testifying, in effect, for the defence, countered by psychiatrists testifying for the other side. It follows that, these psychiatric teams having been selected for their disagreement, the most widely publicized utterances of psychiatrists are usually totally at variance. Sometimes the psychiatrists on one side, usually the defence (which is entitled to go to greater lengths to bolster its case), are obvious to their colleagues as eccentric or heterodox, but the ring of their opinions and the effect of their professional presence may match those of the psychiatrists who find themselves in opposition, so that the respective merits of the differing opinions, which if known would make the controversy unreal, do not become apparent in court.

Once in the witness-box the psychiatrist finds himself in a new role. Accustomed to being tacitly in charge, umpiring the game and changing the rules as he goes along, he is suddenly bound by rigid legal rules of testimony. He may, if he is unfortunate, be subjected to public rudeness for which his training in tolerating private digs has not prepared him. His views are likely to be attacked. He may be asked hypothetical questions of stupefying absurdity and if the circumstances hypothesized are not absolutely impossible, he must answer them. If the person about whom he is testifying is his patient, which is to say that he did not originally see him as a consequence of legal proceedings, he may find himself bound to answer questions that seek to reveal confidential matters. If all these things are liable to happen after the eminent psychiatrist has spent hours or days waiting about and the fee he receives is paltry, the explanation of why psychiatrists undertake legal work with some trepidation is complete.

The lawyers, on the other hand, find the psychiatrist less than perfect. The doctor is not usually immediately interested in public welfare; he is accustomed to thinking first of his patient, and takes it as a matter of course that in his daily work he should hear and fail to pass on confessions of all kinds of misdemeanours and crimes. Therefore, though the psychiatrist in court should theoretically be answering questions in a kind of emotional vacuum, he not infrequently adopts a defensive posture if he is one of those who believes that the prisoner is ill, warping his answers to suit his general proposition. Furthermore the psychiatrist is accustomed to trying to describe things as they are, in the realization that even the best use of words is imperfect, and he is intolerant of the restrictions the court may place on the way he answers questions. He may believe that his way is best, and show no patience for the legal traditions; by doing so he affronts the court for, despite the near-psychotic schism between evidence presented in court about an event and what actually happened, lawyers are sentimentally attached to their methods.

Some reforms are obviously overdue, for the ones who suffer from imperfections in the system are both the prisoners and the public. In the United States some courts have psychiatric clinics attached or court psychiatrists available. The oldest of these clinics have been in operation for more than thirty years and are highly experienced in the work. At some, for example, Cook County Clinic, Illinois, the defendant must request any psychiatric examination that is done; at others, the court may or must order it. The court thus obtains the opinion of a psychiatrist whose value they have been able to assess over a period and a measure of the confidence they place in familiar opinions may be judged from the fact that where these court clinics exist it is unusual for the defence to call in outside psychiatrists. It is the implications of the latter tendency that constitute one of the principal arguments against instituting these court-affiliated psychiatric services in the United Kingdom, for it is felt that to saddle the defence lawyers with a psychiatrist appointed by the court is to restrict their ability to seize every chance of achieving an acquittal, such a restriction being thought undesirable in the United Kingdom. There is probably something to be said for excluding the lunatic fringe of psychiatrists from court by requiring a minimum of training and experience before expert testimony may be offered, but not all the peculiar opinions heard in court come from the most poorly trained; something seems to come over psychiatrists when they get into the witness-box.

It is natural that a psychiatrist writing on this topic should advocate that the process be made easier for the psychiatrists themselves. There is some self-interest in this suggestion, but it would also make it easier for solicitors to obtain truly expert testimony instead of having to take who they can get. There seems no obvious reason why doctors should not be able to know in advance when their testimony would be required, so that they do not have to cancel clinics suddenly, sometimes without enough warning to put the patients off, or wait fretfully for their turn while valuable working time slips by. Also, where official fees are paid these, though they could not be made commensurate with the trouble, should be of such a size that they do not add insult to injury. In many instances psychiatrists find themselves delivering opinions which do not differ importantly from those given by respected colleagues on the other side, and much time is wasted and obscurity conjured up by legal attempts to stress or dismiss the minor disparity. There is a place for agreed reports in criminal trials, thrashed out by the psychiatrists in pre-trial discussion, on which the court could question a member of the psychiatric committee concerned, preferably (to avoid a semblance of the imposition of arbitrary adjudication) one selected by the defence. There seems no reason why psychiatrists, or any other doctors, should have to go to court to swear that documentary records are what they seem, when neither side contests their genuineness.

All doctors should be protected from the device of the hypothetical question: a psychiatrist in court may be asked to imagine a patient with certain delusions and symptoms and, when he has done so, be asked to say how such a person would act under a particular set of circumstances. Questions like these cannot be answered properly and should be ruled out; it is difficult enough to imagine how the patient himself feels without trying to achieve empathy with lawyers' models.

The question of privilege is frequently raised in medical writings on expert evidence. The principal in a trial may avoid the witness-box, his solicitor is protected from questioning by legal rules, and Roman Catholic priests are protected because they may not reveal information received in the confessional, so questioning them about such facts would simply be malicious. No other citizens may keep silent in court without laying themselves open to the unrestricted penalties available to an affronted judge.

Outside the court, doctors maintain confidentiality about their patients. Some patients do not realize that this is so and display some nervousness about material they disclose, while others are more concerned about the possibility of written records finding their way into the wrong hands, but most patients take it for granted that what they say will not be repeated outside a medical setting. Unfortunately, if they are consulting the doctor, in the present instance the psychiatrist, about matters which could ever be brought up in court, they are unwise to make this assumption. At present there is nothing to prevent a spouse who wants a divorce from obtaining the testimony of her husband's psychiatrist, to whom he may have confessed suitable grounds. A psychiatrist seeing a patient for some trait currently regarded as antisocial, such as homosexuality, later might conceivably find his notes adding to a case against his patient. If such a patient is seen because he has been accused, the psychiatrist should warn him that to be frank at the interview will be tantamount to confessing at the trial and that even if the patient has never been accused before and is pleading guilty, great circumspection should be used in talking about previous homosexual conduct lest the helpful fiction of a first offence be destroyed; such warnings make a mockery of the interview.

On the other hand, the importance of the law cannot be

denied, and in their work even the most anarchic psychiatrists pay attention to the law, or to the morality it reflects. Psychiatrists may and do assist a homosexual practising with consenting adults to adjust to this style of life in order that he may be happier, but few or none of them would offer the same facilities to a patient who lusted after children. They would indulge in misprision of a felony already committed by failing to tell the authorities, but would probably intervene if the felony were such as to cause physical harm to others and was still in the planning stage. There are occasions when the course of justice would be violently diverted by the silence of a psychiatrist with key information. The arguments against psychiatric privilege are strong and in this country have so far prevailed.

Reform is not entirely impracticable. In the United States medical privilege is commonplace. Psychiatric privilege, recognized as more necessary because of the peculiarly intimate nature of the communications, is assured by statute in two thirds of the States and by case-law in several more. Where the psychiatrist saw the patient for the purposes of the legal action, privilege does not cover him. In this country psychiatry has not reached the same level of acceptance, but even here the type of questions psychiatrists are supposed to ask is so well known that patients feel cheated if they have not had a grilling about their sex-life, and the inequity of publishing the results of such interviews must be obvious. It ought to be possible to provide for privilege in civil cases, and for some qualified privilege in criminal cases, and a movement is under way to negotiate some such provision for the profession and for the patients who speak frankly of the past.

DIVORCE

In England divorce may be obtained on psychiatric grounds, and psychiatric considerations enter into the assessment of cruelty when this ground is quoted.

A husband or wife may obtain a divorce if the partner has been continuously under care in a recognized psychiatric hospital for five years, and if the condition is considered by experts to be incurable. Obtaining a divorce on the grounds of insanity is a recognized method in many countries, even those where a different public morality allows little opportunity for divorce in most cases. The application of this law makes it possible for the unaffected marital partner to take up life and companionship again, and is in general benign. Over the last ten years its application has been narrowed by changes in treatment and the law. Psychiatrists have become more hesitant about stating that a patient is incurable since despite the intractable nature of the long-standing patients' illnesses as a group, some few improvements of a remarkable degree have taken place under new régimes, particularly at the beginning of the tranquillizer era.

Case-law seems to be establishing, however, that the likelihood that a given patient can be discharged at some time in the future does not of itself refute the proposition that the patient is incurable; it must be stated, for divorce to be prevented, that the patient is not only liable to leave hospital, but will then be able to take up married life again approximately as if no illness had taken place. The other flaw, caused by recent legislation about hospital admissions, and widened by hospital policy, is that many patients become able to leave hospital if they choose, and may, by doing so for more than a month, interrupt the continuity on which the petitioner relies. Some modification of this statute is therefore required, if, as is likely, the grounds themselves are still thought adequate.

An alternative method of obtaining a divorce is to plead that the spouse who became a patient was cruel. Until recently the M'Naughton rules, of which more will be said later, were held to apply so that if the cruel conduct arose out of delusional ideas the offending spouse was held not to be responsible for the conduct and divorce was refused. A decision delivered by the House of Lords in 1963 now makes it clear that the courts will give a decree essentially on the basis of the gravity of the conduct; this decision making divorce much easier to obtain, a tendency with which psychiatrists, in common with many of their social class, are in sympathy especially now that obtaining divorce on the simple grounds of incurable insanity is becoming less practicable.

In Scotland alcoholism is taken of itself to constitute cruelty and thus provides a ground for divorce; in England this equivalence is not allowed and the matter must be proved separately. In this, as in other aspects of the law, Scotland is probably ahead of England. Much hardship might be avoided by bringing the statutes into line on both sides of the border.

ABORTION

Therapeutic abortion may be advised if the mother's life is threatened by the pregnancy or, as has come to be allowed, if continuation of the pregnancy would make the mother a mental or physical wreck. The physical diseases which, if present, make abortion sometimes advisable, are less frequently found today or less seriously regarded. The incidence of therapeutic abortion on psychiatric grounds is increasing, however, and the reasons for this arise out of the ease with which psychiatrists can be made to see the necessity for the operation.

In certain instances the mother-to-be should be aborted if her health is to be considered responsibly. Intervention in the pregnancy of a patient who has had a severe schizophrenic illness with a long course, precipitated by a previous delivery and followed by an only just adequate recovery, may spare her from the risk of further post-schizophrenic defect. The patient with many children and more problems, living in precarious equilibrium and permanently on the point of moral collapse, may be kept going by restricting her brood. In both the instances mentioned, simultaneous sterilization might be considered, but not if the woman had a chance of fresh marital partners. Apart from the (small) immediate risks of abortion, there is the possibility that the puerperal psychosis that was to be prevented will be precipitated by the miniature delivery that is done, and the probability that the patient will experience guilt at a later time about her part in the operation. Sterilization, advisedly undertaken, seems to cause little or no upset.

In most cases, however, the abortion is recommended on the grounds that the patient's life is in danger from suicide. She is thought to be depressed and she states that if the pregnancy continues she will kill herself. These *prima facie* grounds do not usually bear close examination: if she is depressed enough to kill herself she needs admission to a good hospital, not an operation; and coroner's records show that the suicide of a pregnant woman is an event of extreme rarity.

As in other dealings with the law, doctors take on the role of accomplice (kindly called, in a recent article 'the unwitting accomplice'), counselling abortion because they think the law ought to allow it to be performed under wider conditions than statutorily prevail, and often their real reason for the operation is a feeling of sympathy, a feeling which may be more easily aroused in the case of spinsters if the patients concerned come from their own social class.

COMPENSATION NEUROSIS

Patients who have sustained injuries – particularly mild injuries – in industrial accidents are liable to develop neurotic disabilities of an incapacitating type. Compensation is assessed on the basis of current disability and its prognosis, and the question of the outlook for this type of neurosis is therefore one of some medico-legal importance. It was not known until recently whether the lost function and well-being returned after settlement of the claim, and psychiatric reservations about the facile assumption that this would occur were reflected in the size of the awards given. It is now known with certainty that compensation or traumatic neurosis clears up when the case is settled, and that unless a case is pending it does not occur. Reduction in morbidity therefore awaits speeding up of the legal processes, and in order to eradicate the condition a change in the law relating to industrial compensation is needed.

SEXUAL CRIMES

If the number of offences known to the police is taken as a guide, and poor though it is there is no better, the amount of criminal sexual behaviour that takes place in the United Kingdom has risen greatly (about threefold) over the last generation and has done so at an even higher rate than other crimes. The level of recorded crime bears more relationship to such chance factors as local police policy, methods of recording and charging, current fashions in prudery (whether these prevent or encourage complaints), and so on than to how many misdemeanours have actually taken place. But though some auxiliary evidence, such as that provided by Kinsey's surveys, seems to show that in sexual matters things stay about the same from generation to generation with little difference in tastes or their gratification, and while the occurrence of illegitimacy, which has halved over the last century, might indicate a certain increase in sexual restraint, the incidence of rape has also been rising so that the higher incidence of sexual crimes cannot be dismissed as entirely an artefact.

Proportionately, sexual crimes form a small part – 2 or 3 per cent – of the indictable offences known to have taken place. About 80 per cent are cleared up, compared with about 40 per cent for other crime and less than 20 per cent for wage-snatches, but the factor of being caught in the act is the most important in this degree of success; where no offence is observed detection of the offender is difficult, and while officially determined sexual recidivism is infrequently found the number of habitual sexual offenders who are never prosecuted is, taking the whole range of offences, very high; for example, only a very few adults are charged with homosexual activity in private with a consenting adult, though hundreds of thousands of felonious homosexual offences of this kind must take place weekly in this country.

Psychiatric interest in sexual offences is restricted to the phenomenology of the perversions and the diagnosis of incidentally associated mental abnormality, but psychiatrists are frequently called in to examine sexual offenders either because the magistrate finds the conduct so incomprehensible as to smack of psychological imbalance or because the accused wishes to cast a protective mantle about himself.

The perversions themselves are, though interesting, difficult to plead in mitigation; if people did not have a taste for certain forbidden acts they would not be forbidden, and the fact that the taste is ingrained does not make it less culpable. Nevertheless though, like the personality disorders they are allied to, the perversions are described rather than diagnosed, naming them has come to count as a diagnosis and many psychiatrists are willing to state that an accused person is, for example, a homosexual and that treatment can be undertaken, because they are in favour of softening the laws of the age.

In fact, perverted patients are those whose sexual tastes are seldom entirely novel and are only quantitatively different from those of the majority. Discussion of the question of penalties for sexual offences often generates a fair amount of rancour – probably because even the 'normal' are half-aware of a modicum of perversion in themselves. It is generally thought that the best known of the perversions, homosexuality, is a trait that follows a normal (or gaussian) distribution (with heterosexuality at the opposite pole) corresponding to that of intelligence and height. Even with such an uncommon perversion as fetishism, in which a neutral or non-genital object replaces the female and her genitalia as the target of sexual desire, the seed of the abnormality may be said to exist in those of us who admire particular aspects of a woman preferentially, and to have germinated in those who insist on certain forms of dress or display in their wives.

The author is approaching, in a roundabout way, the proposition that what is illegal is not necessarily abnormal and, in addition to this, that most perversions as such do not constitute psychiatric illnesses. Perversions may cause much misery and even ruin to the unfortunates who suffer them, whether continently or incontinently, but their principal effects on the individual concerned are the consequence of their illegality or the feelings of guilt they inspire, particularly the former. To illustrate this point: it is common to see adult males complaining solely of their homosexual propensities, which are illegal, but uncommon to the point of rarity to see adult females complaining of theirs, which are not.

As for the first proposition, that what is illegal is not necessarily abnormal, the crime of indecent assault against girls under sixteen, which is taken to occur even if the girl gives her full consent and requires for its completion no more than physical contact of a sexually intended kind, would, if invariably discovered and regularly prosecuted, result in the wholesale punishment and incarceration for recidivism of the healthiest and the most outward bound of our youth.

Because psychiatrists disapprove of many of the sexual laws and their chancy use, they consent to the faulty supposition that they have something medical to offer persons who are charged, and speak up in court about the pitiable nature of the infliction and the hopes that the patient, though he cannot help himself, may respond to certain measures, to be decided later after fuller investigation. Their advice is usually accepted. Psychiatrists are notably less willing to say as much in defence of those who molest children, though *medically* the essence of the matter is very similar, and the fact is that in cases involving perversion, as in many others, the psychiatrist is acting less like a doctor than a liberal citizen who sees an opportunity of intervening in a threatened injustice.

Exploitation of the same general misconceptions as prevail in court enables social protection to be provided for perverts who undergo social disapproval, either following or separate from legal action, and the patient (as he nominally becomes) and his relatives and circle are provided with a medical tag and the outward trappings of treatment. The sharp divergence of aims between the lawyers (who require evidence of illness before they will allow extenuation) and the psychiatrists (who blithely produce straightforward descriptions as if they were speaking of diseases because they wish to see no penalty imposed) makes for most of the confusion about the subject as it is displayed in court, especially since the divergence is for obvious reasons seldom made explicit unless the psychiatrist disapproves of the sexual conduct with which the man is charged.

Public concern is aroused by those whose sexual activities involve children and by recidivists, particularly if the latter are child-molesters. Misconceptions exist; it is sometimes said that the homosexual recidivist undergoes a kind of degeneration, undertaking felonious conduct with younger and younger partners until at last he resorts to boys, and a similar view exists of the progressive style of heterosexual paedophiliacs – who have been suspected of performing more and more serious offences on small girls. In fact, it seems that neither homosexual nor heterosexual recidivists change their style over the years.

Psychiatrists cannot assist the courts in the management of these, the most antisocial of the sexual recidivists, except by making it clear that they have no certain or permanent means of protecting the public and that, if the court is considering separating the accused from those he menaces, no expectation exists that time or treatment will alter him. Corrective measures, in the reformative sense, are even more unlikely to work with paedophiliac recidivists than with most criminals since a high proportion of this group are self-indulgent psychopaths with alternative sexual outlets, previous records of non-sexual crime, and a grand capacity for self-deception and self-justification, while a higher proportion of dullards is found in this than in most other groups of offenders.

Notwithstanding what has been said so far about the importance of medical practitioners in this area of human conduct, there is one set of measures that is sometimes used, with qualified success. Though the direction of desire cannot be altered in the vast majority of the patients seen and continence cannot be influenced by exhortation where punishment fails, the level of sexual desire can be reduced by certain measures, as the proprietors of harems knew many centuries ago. Castration is legally performed on sexual recidivists in certain countries, notably some States in America and Scandinavian countries, where the procedure is thinly disguised as voluntary though the operational reason the prisoner has for agreeing is that he will thereby reduce his penalty. Fortunately there is no prospect of this measure gaining ground here, but what might be termed medical castration is sometimes used; it is possible, by administering female sex hormones to a male, temporarily to reduce libido to the point where perverts, particularly those with a socially acceptable sexual outlet as well as the forbidden one, can control their weakened urges to transgress. A convicted sexual offender may be put on probation on condition he follows medical advice (for a maximum of one year) and during this period of enforced cooperation he can be treated, to use the conventional term, with these suppressive agents. In these instances, as with surgical castration, the subjects indicate that they equate the measures with punishment (by stopping the drug at the end of the term no matter what they may have said on the topic of remorse) and usually, perhaps always, return to their old pleasures, showing how hard it is to work against the intense rewards which deviants gain from the sexual activity of their preference.

The laws relating to sexual conduct, more so than most others, are in urgent need of reform. A psychiatrist is not necessarily more expert at suggesting the manner in which they should be changed than the criminal psychologist or the sociologist, but some unsatisfactory aspects of the laws cry out for alteration. Overall the laws should bear some relationship to reality; people do indulge their tastes, whether perverted or not, and are not responsible for more than a proportion of their incontinence, which depends more notably on the level of innate sexual drive than the individual's self-control. Correspondingly, the 'dark figure' – the numbers of crimes committed but never reported – is gigantic in the sexual field, greater even, it might be, than the dark figures for drunk driving or speeding.

If laws are not going to be enforced they should be dropped; the aphorism that bad laws should be enforced (in order that their injustice might be highlighted by a martyr or two) does not seem to apply to sexual (and particularly homosexual) crime, where there have been martyrs aplenty, but the urge to punish among the unthinking public strung along the gaussian curve is great and irrational, and persists despite shame at vicious penalties distributed by lot. The failure to alter laws referring to perverted conduct committed in private between consenting adults is a blot on democracy that is not expunged by the more liberal prosecution policy that has been introduced privately by politicians too self-interested to speak up in public.

Heterosexual activity of an otherwise normal kind is penalized if it occurs outside certain stipulated ages. It is in general illegal for any sexual activity to be permitted with a girl under the age

of sixteen, though if the young man concerned is himself inexperienced and the girl looks and says she is of the age of
consent a defence of ignorance may be raised. Now few would
disagree that the young girl, like the young boy, should be
protected from the wiles of older men; but girls of less than
sixteen do indulge in sexual play with their male contemporaries
and as recent articles in newspapers (together with memories of
individual adolescences) indicate, many seek and welcome sexual
intercourse. The early maturation of young people today and
the possibly greater tendency to experience sexual activity
should receive statutory recognition; the policy relating to
prosecution is liberal, but remains too capricious, as even
slight inconsistency must where maximum penalties are high.

All in all, and accepting that the view taken of sexual offences
may be a restricted one, it does not seem necessary to forbid
what adults do in private or penalize heavily what many do by
mutual consent. If the heavy penalties were restricted to those
whose conduct caused actual or probable harm (bodily or
psychological) to their partners, psychiatrists would be called
less often, would rarely be able to give testimony in mitigation,
and the confusion would be less. Reforms have been proposed
that would remove the necessity for the victim, if a child, to
attend the court to give evidence, but it is doubtful if depositions
by a child, immune from gentle cross-examination, could serve
the course of justice; the author believes, with Kinsey, that
some allegations are malicious or unfounded. But, reviewing the
survey they made, the Cambridge Department of Criminal
Science admitted that 'after investigating more than 3,000 cases
the Department is no nearer to a constructive recommendation
for the general treatment of sexual offenders than it was when it
began its inquiries'.

MURDER

Murderers are the criminal group whose psychiatric disabilities are the most obvious; 50 per cent of murderers are
insane and about 20 per cent commit suicide before the law can
take its course; apart from the murder he commits, the indi-

vidual is not usually concerned in major crime. Our knowledge of murderers is incomplete, partly at least because of the promptness with which even the most normal of them were dispatched, but the very existence of the death penalty has made for considerable interest in the psychiatric states of those accused or awaiting execution, and despite the artificial nature of interviews conducted under these abnormal circumstances a certain amount of recorded clinical material is available to the researcher.

In pre-trial work it has been the task of the psychiatrist, until recent years, to determine the patient's mental state with particular reference to the M'Naughton rules. These rules have dominated the medico-legal aspect of major crime, notably murder, for more than a hundred years, and apart from their now limited applicability in this country are the sole test of criminal responsibility in twenty-nine of the United States and much of the Commonwealth. The subject of M'Naughton has been written about very often in the last few years, and received a fairly full treatment in newspapers whenever the defence called for a verdict of guilty but insane in a prominent murder trial, so that the nature and significance of M'Naughton will be explained only briefly.

In the early nineteenth century there were a series of murders or attempted assassinations of royalty committed by subjects who were clearly mentally abnormal. The requirement that a citizen had to be so mad and devoid of reason as to be akin to a beast before criminal responsibility could be shrugged off was already effectively defunct, and the general ruling was based on a notion, then popular, that insanity could be incomplete, with retention of reason in some spheres and loss of it in others. Superficially, certain patients, particularly well-preserved paranoid patients with systematized delusions of long standing, can certainly appear rational enough when discussing neutral matters and can employ normal logic when drawing inter-mediate conclusions in their delusional arguments.

On the assumption that partial insanity of this kind could exist, the tendency was to require that the defence connected the act committed with the insane element in the patient, which meant in effect that the jury had to be satisfied that the delusion led directly to the act. In the decades before M'Naughton the juries in the famous trials were told what the consequences of finding the prisoner not guilty on the grounds of insanity (as the verdict was then) would be – detention until the King's pleasure should be known – and despite the treasonable nature of some of the offences committed the juries were rather liberal in their verdicts. No clear rulings existed for the guidance of the courts, however, and there was a certain unevenness in the application of the law, escape from the supreme penalty depending on the excellence of the counsel provided in treason trials rather than the application of clear precedents.

The unsatisfactory state of the law was brought to public attention when, in 1843, a paranoid schizophrenic called Daniel M'Naughton shot and killed the Prime Minister's secretary in mistake for Sir Robert Peel himself. In the subsequent trial M'Naughton was shown by the prosecution to be entirely capable of conducting certain business matters, including buying firearms for the deed, in a sensible and forthright manner, while the defence showed him to be so deluded and persecuted in his mind as to be probably unfit to plead by the standards of the present day. By concentrating on the partial insanity of the patient and the relevance of his delusional system to the murderous act, counsel for the defence so influenced the court as to lead to the case being stopped with the prisoner found not guilty because of his insanity.

Though the finding was incontestable and served the cause of common humanity the uncertain state of the law was a source of disturbance both for the public and the legislature. Therefore the Lords consulted the judges, in a legally hallowed manner, by putting questions to them about how the law stood and how it might properly be stated. Almost unanimously the judges answered, *inter alia*, that the accused would be punishable if it could not 'be clearly proved, that, at the time of the committing of the act, the party accused was labouring under such a defect of reason, from disease of the mind, as not to know the nature and quality of the act he was doing, or, if he did know it, that he did not know he was doing what was wrong'. Furthermore, if the accused laboured under delusions with respect only to limited aspects of his total ideation, 'he must be considered in the same situation as to responsibility as if the facts with respect to which the delusion exists were real. For example, if, under the influence of his delusion, he supposes another man to be in the act of attempting to take away his life, and he kills that man, as he supposes, in self-defence, he would be exempt from punishment. If his delusion was that the deceased had inflicted a serious injury to his character and fortune, and he killed him in revenge for such supposed injury, he would be liable to punishment.'

Evidently, few parties so disordered that they did not know the nature and quality of the act or, if they knew it, did not know it was wrong (meaning wrong in law, in effect), are fit to plead and in recent years the legal arguments have centred around the necessity of demonstrating that the accused party's delusions were not only such that they might have made him angry or aggrieved but such that they would have made his act justifiable homicide had they been true. The strict application of these rules would have debarred all but a few murderers, even obviously psychotic murderers, from clemency, but the main arguments against their application lay not in their intrinsic injustice, which the juries forestalled by refusing to convict if the accused was obviously psychiatrically ill, but in the capricious manner in which they were enforced and the way in which the rules persisted long after psychiatric advances had confirmed the falseness of the assumptions about partial insanity on which they were based.

Nineteenth-century psychiatrists who were interested in jurisprudence wrote critical commentaries on the rules, and though the M'Naughton rules were widely accepted by many states and countries during the years after their formal expression, there were other sets of rules in force to which reformers could look for support. It was established in the nineteenth century in New Hampshire that what was required of their defence lawyers was that they should show that the act was in some comprehensible way the 'product' of the mental illness from which the patient suffered. In Scotland also it was rightly supposed that the existence of delusions was enough to make it doubtful whether the close logic required of the patient by the M'Naughton rules could really be supposed to be available to the mind of the accused. Psychiatrists giving expert testimony found that questions and answers had to conform to the outdated M'Naughton psychopathology, so that such assistance as they might have been able to give was artificially curtailed, a state of affairs that they criticized more frequently as time went by. In practice the M'Naughton rules proved adequate only because they were circumvented.

Many psychotic patients never came to trial. Others were found guilty but insane without the prosecution or judge attempting to apply the rules with any rigour. In closely argued cases the jury would find the accused guilty but insane if it seemed sensible to do so, without regard to the wording of the rules, unless the crime committed were especially repugnant. Even for those murderers whose mental state had not protected them from the pronouncement of the death penalty there were post-trial inquiries, increasingly more liberal as the years went by, whose committee could recommend that execution be replaced by indefinite detention – the Queen's pleasure.

In the nineteen-fifties various movements directed against the frequent imposition of the death penalty became influential. The campaign against the death penalty in this country succeeded in pricking the Government into appointing a Royal Commission on Capital Punishment and the M'Naughton rules were criticized by various bodies during the tendering of evidence. In 1957 in the United States the District of Columbia adopted a rule similar to the old 'product' rule of New Hampshire. The arguments that the relaxation of M'Naughton would lead to a spate of murders with feigned insanity by the murderers faded away with the arguments that the abandonment of the death penalty itself would lead to a wave of murder, countries without capital punishment finding no evidence for this belief. The time was ripe for abandonment of the death penalty, or, failing that, for revision of M'Naughton. The Government decided that the abolition of capital punishment would be premature because it was in advance of the will of the people, though perhaps it was no more so than many reforms done in the past.

The Royal Commission's recommendations that henceforth the degree of insanity should be displayed at the trial to the jury and that the jury should then decide on the matter of whether non-responsibility had been proved, was rejected. Instead of making a bold choice the Homicide Act (1957) was passed. This is a very poor piece of legislation, comfortably regarded by psychiatrists and many others as a passing phase – though M'Naughton has seemed temporary for a disquietingly long time. The Homicide Act goes part of the way towards abolishing capital punishment, selecting only certain types of murder for the death penalty – less than 20 per cent of the whole. Because criminals of all types prefer jail, which they have heard about and are familiar with, to Broadmoor, the scope of M'Naughton is greatly reduced by the circumspection of capital murder, a defence of insanity being used only uncommonly in non-capital murder cases. Furthermore, though clear-cut insanity still provides a separate form of defence, the Act introduces, with more sense than was applied to its division of murders into capital and non-capital categories, the concept of 'diminished responsibility'.

This idea – that degrees of mental disorder less profound than outright psychosis can affect such factors as a person's self-control – is an old one in law and is, of course, in accordance with common experience; in Scotland a similar doctrine has been in operation for a long while, and in other countries including some American States the defence of 'irresistible impulse', meaning some failure of self-control, may sometimes be raised. The Homicide Act (1957, Section 2) states that 'where a person kills or is a party to the killing of another, he shall not be convicted of murder if he was suffering from such abnormality of mind (whether arising from a condition of arrested or retarded development of mind or any inherent development of mind or any inherent causes or induced by disease or injury) as substantially impaired his mental responsibility for his acts and omissions in doing or being a party to the killing'. The onus of proof lies on the defence, and if the defence carries the point with the jury, a verdict of manslaughter is returned instead of murder; if the defence overshoots and shows that the accused is insane the jury may still return a verdict of guilty but insane if they choose.

The provision for 'diminished responsibility' marks not only a departure from the strict requirements of M'Naughton for those who are insane but allows the inclusion of psychopaths. The law recognizes that this troublesome group is marked by evidence of failures of self-control and includes them, for this purpose, with those who suffer similar ill-defined and quantitative defects – such as the high-grade mental defective who might also (but does not necessarily) qualify for inclusion – as well as those who are definitely, though perhaps mildly, psychiatrically ill.

The difference between psychopath and psychotic is that the psychotic displays definite failures in one or more compartments of activity as well as some overall falling off in efficiency, and can be said to suffer from a precise type of impairment; while the psychopath is adjudged different from those around him only because he behaves in general in an unfortunate or feckless or irresponsible (but not an odd or bizarre) way. Psychotic patients are a medical responsibility because they suffer from illness, and are accepted as patients whether or not something can be done for them; nobody disagrees that their responsibility for their overall conduct is impaired. The psychopath, on the other hand, is really accepted for treatment not because of the illness he shows, since he shows none, but because the psychiatrist, having some knowledge of psychology and a willingness to help, can often provide some assistance, mainly of an advisory kind, to the patient; he assists because he is able in a limited way to do so, calls what he does 'treatment' out of habit, calls the psychopath a 'patient' because he is accustomed to label his clients in this way, and calls psychopathy a diagnosis because most of the labels he attaches are diagnoses and it does not occur to him to except this one. But it should be stressed that he does not treat the psychopath in the usual medical way and he diagnoses no disease; the psychopath's responsibility for his conduct, in so far as this conception can be applied to the activities of others, is complete.

What is happening then? The new law, imperfect but better than those that went before, is guilty of mixing its motives. It reduces the extent to which capital punishment may be applied; it takes the sting out of M'Naughton; and at the same time it introduces a new mitigating quasi-medical condition, effectively that of psychopathy, that is welcomed by psychiatrists despite its illogicality. It seems that this law is a casualty of compromise. In so far as it moved towards the abolition of capital punishment it was welcomed by many, including perhaps the majority of psychiatrists, on emotional grounds; on the same grounds, the main criticisms directed against it were connected with the remnant of capital murders. But regarded in the cold light of reason it is crazy that a man should be able to plead that his long career of wrongdoing makes it obvious that he is suffering from an abnormality of mind sufficient to reduce his crime to manslaughter while another, previously innocent of crime but in all other respects identical, should hang. It is as if there was an abolitionist reformer among the committee who drafted the act, who infiltrated as many escape clauses as he could without regard to their logical justification (and probably this was what actually happened).

The subject of psychopathy is dealt with elsewhere, and the provision for psychopaths in other psychiatric legislation discussed later in the next chapter; the topic is one on which much confused discussion has focused, but it is not the nature of psychopathy or psychoticism or sin that makes the Homicide Act, M'Naughton and questions of impaired responsibility so vexing and confused; it is capital punishment. Without the death penalty the law would suddenly become lucid and simple, as it has done in non-capital murder. No reform but abolition need seriously be recommended.

OTHER CRIMES

The statistically normal nature of crime should once again be stressed: many or most citizens have committed crimes, and most are not brought to book. Psychiatrists may pontificate but they do not know about the roots of crime, and the study of the

80 per cent of criminals who show no psychiatric abnormality at all – the 'normal criminals' – is not one that they can or should claim as their own. They can diagnose psychiatric conditions in a few per cent of the criminals they see, and treat or intervene to prevent punishment, and they occasionally accept responsibility for the management of the psychopathic (often called sociopathic in this context) criminal, particularly if his main flaw seems to be immaturity rather than callousness. They may point out the importance of biographical events in the life of an accused if these are of such a nature as to show why the man, through no fault of his own, has a different view of society from the judge. They may indicate how even small changes of personality such as those seen in women before menstruation (at which time they commit most of their crimes, particularly their few crimes of violence) can alter the liability to offend. But for the most part, in spite of occasional claims to the contrary, the psychiatrist stands on the sidelines and has little constructive to say. His training does not equip him for, and his treatment does not assist him in, the management of a qualitively normal group.

TREATMENT OF THE OFFENDER

The phrase 'treatment of the offender', now in general use, indicates how far the idea of the criminal as a sick victim of genes and environment has caught on. Strictly speaking, treatment should presumably be given only to those who are suffering from a recognized illness or, taking a broader catchment, who have mental states that would qualify them, without regard to their criminality as such, for management by a doctor. As it is used in sociological work, treatment refers to what used to be called corrective measures, including those whose most obvious characteristic is punitive, and part of the justification for using it instead of the old-fashioned word 'punishment' is that some of the techniques of psychiatry are being transplanted to the prisons.

The methods used to deal with the offender in the past, and at the present time, are intended to be retributive, along the lines of an eye for an eye; segregational, so that the criminal is kept away from trouble; deterrent, so that he hesitates to do it again; and corrective, so that he does not want to.

Retribution is now exacted less fiercely and the severity of penalties has decreased markedly over the years, even where the statutory maxima for the crimes have not been altered. The long-term segregation of incorrigibles is being done more frequently and many countries now have recidivist statutes, allowing preventive detention or its equivalent when all other measures have failed to induce reform and the crimes are serious enough to affront or damage the public. Though no doubt justifiable, this type of measure is born of despair.

The deterrent aspect of punishment, when it achieves publicity, is aimed partly at potential criminals in the expectation that they will reject thoughts of wrongdoing. Otherwise, the deterrent or corrective measures are intended to affect the criminal himself, reducing his propensity for crime.

In this country 75 per cent of first offenders do not come before a court on a criminal charge again, regardless of the punishment meted out, and there is anecdotal evidence that even the fright produced by a charge without a conviction frequently causes a change of heart. 'Relapse' does not apparently depend on what type of punishment was used, even if it was apparently solely aimed at correction – such as the use of probation or psychiatric agencies.

The problem may be expressed thus: the prison population and the level of reported crime is increasing steadily and alarmingly, with about 30,000 now lying in prisons and borstals. Though about 40 per cent of reported crime is cleared up in this country, the percentage is not high enough for mild punishments to deter with anything approaching the effectiveness they would attain if the proportion was, say 90 per cent. The use of harsh punishments such as those of the nineteenth century, the imposition of which meant not only the horrors of prison for the man but the rigours of the poor law for his family, will not be reintroduced.

The guilty man's future conduct can therefore be most hopefully influenced by corrective measures. If those in use at present were effective to any real extent we should expect to find that some worked better than others. The finding that they all are associated with the same proportion of failures and successes, allowing as far as possible for the other variables, means either that they are all coincidentally of equal usefulness or, as is more probable, that none of them works at all. Therefore new measures are needed, and the experience of psychiatrists who have the reputation of being able to modify pathological conduct, here equated with the socially pathological conduct (speaking metaphorically) called crime is drawn upon where possible.

Because of the non-pathological nature of crime, the methods used by psychiatrists in the treatment of those who are formally ill cannot be applied. But experience with psychopaths enables psychiatrists to offer some expert advice on the manner in which those who find it hard to conform to group requirements can be educated and trained to do so. These methods are not singularly successful in the management of non-criminal personalities, where motivation is high and cooperation automatically assured by the patient's presence, and certain characteristics of the methods themselves make them difficult to apply to prison populations without considerable modification and, it is to be feared, loss of effectiveness.

The patient with a severe personality problem, especially one involving difficulty in conforming, in seeing the point of view of those he upsets, and in learning from experience, can be assisted in a variety of ways, of which the most effective and well known depends on his incorporation within a therapeutic community. The characteristics of such a group should include voluntary participation, self-imposed rules, self-imposed punishments, simplicity of formal organization, absence of hierarchy, and absolute overall fairness. A member is obliged to cooperate in the laying down of simple rules, their manner of formation making them voluntarily acceptable. These rules are preferably so basic that any transgression is known at once, and they cannot be broken without the certainty or near-certainty of discovery. The punishments, usually involving withdrawal of privileges, are fair and firm; they too are self-imposed. All members of the group are equal and the doctors participating avoid as far as possible the accoutrements of professional status so that they do not appear to be in authority – and indeed the control exerted over this type of group is intended to be minimal. Free discussion of such traits as the patients have are conducted at sessions during which, among other things, the cause of failures to conform are analysed.

The dynamics and *modus operandi* of these therapeutic groups can be variously described, but we have as yet no entirely satisfactory way of categorizing the inter-reactions of the participants. It is probably best to regard the group, for the purposes of elucidation, as a powerful learning device, the subject taught being social conformity. The patient has only a few fair rules to follow, against which rebellion is as difficult to justify as would be the peremptory refusal of goods one has examined, ordered, and paid for. Punishment is certain, swift, and as just, at the least, as the punishment the patient himself has participated in administering.

Refuge in lack of insight and rationalization of an initially conscious kind is prevented by the insights of the group which, even if they are wrong in detail, are likely to bring home to the patient his own motivations and the inappropriateness of his conduct in the setting. The patient finds himself living in a kind of idealized world, where social contacts occur at a feverishly high rate and failure is greeted with sympathy and does not lead to long-standing withdrawal of approval or entries in a dossier. Being someone who is slow to learn the rules of the world, he is given an opportunity of picking them up at leisure.

In prisons, group psychotherapy is one of the major innovations of the past decade. Evidently, it may resemble that done in the therapeutic communities for patients with disordered personalities more in its outward appearance than in its dynamic structure and true parameters. Non-criminal patients with personality disorders seek treatment because their conduct has ultimately produced unhappiness for them and looks like doing so inevitably unless it alters. Criminals have treatment thrust upon them though their conduct produced unhappiness only because they were caught, the chances of their being caught again for any future single criminal act being rather low.

The hospital patients commonly talk of the general organization of the institution in a critical manner and, in the few units that exist, can alter or modify such parts as impinge on them within the limits set by obvious practical considerations. Prisoners' discussions, on the other hand, are not allowed to degenerate into discussions of reform, presumably because of the indiscipline that might follow, though the prisons, as corrective institutions, are patently in great need of reform and it is the experience of those who have conducted group therapy that commonplace topics of this type have to be got out of the way before serious work on psychopathology and interpretation can start. In hospitals, also, the finding is that the more nearly normal the individual members of the group, the less the direction that the doctors should give (a general principle that varies in its application with the personalities and training of particular therapists). Prisoners, a more normal group than even the most mildly afflicted hospital in-patients, are commonly directed more closely than chronic psychotics. The hospital patient is highly motivated towards cure because his aberrant behaviour makes it impossible to realize his intellectual and economic potential. The prisoner is, to be frank, liable to lose money by going straight.

Nevertheless, techniques of persuasion and group pressuring have a place in the management of the normal criminal. They will be more likely to succeed when the severity of punishment for a given offence is less of a lottery, when the prison rules are more humane and reasonable and can therefore be opened for critical consideration (usually a prerequisite for reform), and when the length of the sentence depends, by the availability of suspension, on the progress made by the prisoner. These arrangements would be difficult to fit into the existing judicial and penal systems, and so must depend for most of their successes on the individual personalities of the therapists and prison officers concerned. They are not fanciful arrangements, however, for they have been tried in one form or another in various parts of the world, notably at Herstedvester, in Denmark. In the United States similar methods have been used for the management of sexual offenders, with indefinite imprisonment for psychiatric treatment, release following satisfactory therapeutic progress; and the result was a rather low percentage of (sexual) violation of parole. Corresponding provisions exist for non-sexual and sexual recidivists in Maryland, though it is necessary to convict in that State before compulsory detention can be imposed: those labelled 'defective delinquents' go indefinitely to the Patuxent Institute, where they may stay for life but usually work towards discharge.

The introduction of psychiatry into the jails, both by psychiatric attendances and the new requirement that prison medical officers should have some psychiatric training, means that the one prisoner in five who has some psychiatric condition (including psychopathy) will one day stand a chance of receiving appropriate treatment. It is hard to resist the temptation to be acid about the present standards of care in these uniquely unfair and anti-corrective institutions: perhaps it is sufficient merely to record that in our prisons the strait-jacket, *totally unknown* elsewhere, is still in regular use. Thus, despite disavowals of the primacy of psychiatry in the management of criminals, I think there is room in the jails for much more psychiatric care than is at present provided, and I would suppose that the provision of a therapeutic atmosphere for even a proportion of the inmates would soon lead to changes in the management of the other, normal criminals.

The Law Relating to
15 Psychiatric Patients

It is probably not unjustifiably complacent to believe that the manner in which people are handled by official administrators is on the whole gentler now than at any time in the past. Some unexplained, and to many minds incomprehensible, departures from this humane trend have occurred, notably in Germany a generation ago, but there is ample evidence that many of the punitive and so-called 'charitable' measures of the last century were barbarous and vicious compared with modern usage. For example, prisoners no longer have to turn and toe the wall if an official passes them in the jail corridor, heads are not shaved, and the broad arrow is not worn.

When money is given out to those in need, the nineteenth-century assumption that unless rigorous supervision were undertaken the money would be spent on beer or used to enable the recipient to avoid honest labour is replaced by new but accurate assumptions that cheating is uncommon and the work-shy are rare. It is now possible, in general, to be dependent and in various social and medical difficulties without loss of dignity. It is hard to know quite how this fortunate change has come about, though it is doubtless associated with the increased wealth of the populace and the gradual socialization of most of the services upon which the poor and the sick depend.

The result is greater sympathy and liberality among the public, so that reformers nowadays need only point to a large-scale error or omission for some move to be made to remedy it. That this is a new development is shown by the venerable nature of some of the ills being tackled at present; that the serious efforts that are mobilized are often not adequate for the task is shown by the continued existence of such under-privileged groups as the aged poor.

This new spirit has affected psychiatric patients in many ways, not the least of which is the formal expression given to the wishes of the electorate by recent statutes concerning the psychologically disturbed. The most noticeable change in the law has been the reduction in its use: the law is less often invoked at present for the management of psychiatric patients than at any time since the great Acts of the nineteenth century were passed.

For some years the laws relating to hospital have been modified to make this easier and less formal. In 1930, in the United Kingdom, it became possible to enter a mental hospital as a voluntary patient, while, as previously described, some general hospitals nervously introduced the practice of allowing psychiatric in-patients to be admitted to their wards. In the determinedly liberal and forward-looking countries of Scandinavia there has been a great measure of freedom of entry and exit for a long time and in this country there has been a strong professional movement in favour of easy admission and discharge for many years.

Before the appointed day of the Mental Health Act (1959) most patients in mental hospitals in this country had been admitted under some kind of order, with the agreement of a magistrate, the process being known and feared under the name of 'certification'. The presence of the magistrate, the legalistic form of the documents, the central scrutiny of the procedure by the Board of Control, and all the other checks and safeguards were hangovers from the days when the doctors were not so consistent in their quality, personal liberty was but recently hard-won and was regarded with jealous alertness, and the keepers of mental hospitals were popularly known mainly as villains or figures with which to frighten recalcitrant children. Fear of getting shut away in a mental hospital by mistake was, like getting buried when still alive but unable to speak, a common fear – and a subject for literary exercise – of the claustrophobic Victorians.

After the Second World War, when the National Health Scheme centralized control of almost all the hospital services in the United Kingdom, the administrators of the overall arrangements found that they had many hospitals of very varying standards under their control. Furthermore, the worst were all mental hospitals. These new administrators had no reason to suppose that some natural law compelled this disparity, and favoured vigorous improvement of these hospitals. In the course of examining the problem it became clear that the obstacles were not those of material alone; the formal incarceration of the majority of the patients within their walls made for moral difficulties that were as big a bar to the improvement of the hospitals as lack of money.

At the same time, the post-war years saw a change of heart among the thinking public about mental illness. Popularized versions of Freud's ideas had slowly filtered through, leading people to believe that madness could be analysed out of patients who were really not so much mad as maladjusted; the tranquillizers were publicized as cures; leucotomy operations were accepted with awed and qualified approval; science was thought to be conquering insanity, as it had conquered pneumonia and all other illnesses; and every one was geared to the expectation of cure. Readers who have worked through this book uninterruptedly will know that the propaganda had overreached itself, and things were not really so rosy, but psychiatrists, provided that support was forthcoming for humanitarian and medically sound reforms, were not disturbed by that consideration.

In 1954 the Royal Commission on Mental Illness and Mental Deficiency started its work of inquiry into the law relating to psychiatric patients of all kinds, and the evidence it heard was overwhelmingly in favour of the liberalization of the statutes. Its report led directly to the framing of one of the most enlightened acts of all history, the Mental Health Act (1959). For once, favoured by the spirit of the times and the merit of individual members of the Royal Commission, the law in its final form represented a distillation of the most modern and well-informed professional opinion, repealing previous acts and putting in their place an altogether kinder, simpler, and more thoughtful set of statutory rules.

THE MENTAL HEALTH ACT (1959)

Though this Act made it much easier to admit patients compulsorily to psychiatric hospitals, it is intended that the procedures available for this purpose should not be used if at all possible; that patients who refuse to enter hospital should be persuaded to do so; and that patients whose mental state prevents them from expressing any wish should be admitted for their own benefit precisely as an unconscious patient would be admitted to an ordinary hospital bed. Furthermore, any hospital may accept any kind of patient, so that psychiatric patients may go freely to general hospitals, whether informally or under an order (i.e. unwillingly); on the other hand, the existence of an order or recommendation for admission does not statutorily require a hospital to admit a patient, the hospital being entitled to refuse to do so if it is felt that no suitable accommodation or treatment can be offered.

The Act repealed much previous legislation and dissolved the Board of Control. This body, a semi-autonomous committee, had served to inspect hospitals, encourage progress, and protect the interests of patients for most of this century. It had done invaluable work. It was felt that the Ministry of Health could undertake the same functions without loss of benefit to the patients or the level of amenities provided. Though this is possibly true, the dissolution of the independent Board of Control was a matter for some regret. They had done their work well and for many years were one of the main instruments of hospital reform, because they strove to make mental hospitals attain the standards of the best among them. Decentralized control of the hospitals has been vested, from the aspect of patients' rights, in local tribunals, called Mental Health Review Tribunals, and the Act set these up and defined their constitution.

The Act went on to define the terms it used, and it was at this point that the novelty of its approach, predictable from the Report of the Royal Commission which was its basis, was confirmed.

As usual in these acts, various older terms were dropped because of the odium that usage had attached to them. The term 'mental disorder' was introduced as a blanket term to cover mental illness, subnormality, etc., while the terms idiot, imbecile, and moron or feeble-minded (in descending order of severity) were abandoned and in their place the phrases 'Severe subnormality' (subsuming idiot and imbecile) and 'subnormality' (corresponding roughly to feeble-mindedness) were introduced. This process is illogical, but psychologically justifiable; the appellation 'lunatic asylum' is one that literally and etymologically implies no blame and suggests that the sufferer is protected rather than locked away but its connotations became different with time and the profession were glad to see it fall into disuse some years ago.

The Act, having got this out of the way, went on to define a new category of patient, the psychopath – a psychopathic disorder meaning a persistent disorder or disability of mind (whether or not including subnormality of intelligence) which results in abnormally aggressive or seriously irresponsible conduct on the part of the patient and requires or is susceptible to treatment. The inclusion of this group was a realistic departure from previous legislation: these are people who, if they came under the administrative hammer in earlier times, did so almost always for the purpose of punishment. That they did not respond to punishment and seemed in some way unable to act thoughtfully and normally had long caused disquiet, and the Act recognized what the majority of (but not all) psychiatrists accept – that the question was not whether or not they should be punished but what was the best thing to do with them. In the best traditions of a legislature determined not to interfere with private morals, the Act specifically excluded from the ranks of the mentally disordered those whose abnormality consisted solely of promiscuity.

Part I of the Act, then, set out the scene for the main provisions to follow. Parts II and III enjoined local Authorities to set up facilities for looking after the needs of patients residing in their areas and laid down rules for the registration and conduct of nursing homes and private mental hospitals.

Part IV contained the new provisions for compulsory admission. Previous to the present Act, depriving one of Her Majesty's subjects of his liberty had always entailed, within a very few days, obtaining the approval of a magistrate; in the case of the mentally ill he had to convince himself, regardless of medical opinion about diagnosis, that the patient was so severely disturbed as to be a danger to himself or others; it was not enough that a patient showed the early signs of a disease which, if unchecked, would become progressively more difficult – and ultimately impossible – to treat; recent conduct of an alarming nature, obviously meriting at the least an examination and investigation, did not suffice to keep a patient in hospital if his current conduct was within the wide limits of normality recognized by magistrates born into a culture that admires eccentricity.

These requirements, that a non-expert of acknowledged integrity should be the arbiter of liberty and that oddity was not to be penalized, were admirable. There is a fear still that subtle means may be used in the over-organized twentieth-century State to infringe the real liberty of the individual or that governments may attempt to standardize the conduct and attitudes of the masses. There is also a feeling that psychiatrists may regard as abnormal anything that is not obviously wholesome and that therefore almost any quirk could be used as a tag to append to a patient and thereby dispatch him to hospital; and that once in hospital the use of shock treatment drains the individuality until only a husk, normalized but hollow, remains. (Alan Sillitoe, in *The Decline and Fall of Frankie Buller*, wrote: '"What did they give you shock treatment for, Frankie?" I asked this question calmly, genuinely unable to comprehend what he told me, until the full horrible details of what Frankie must have undergone flashed into my mind. And then I wanted power in me to tear down those white-smocked mad interferers with Frankie's coal-forest world, wanted to wipe out their hate and presumption.')

The only excuse for depriving people of their liberty more easily and with less supervision would be if the inquisitorial process of confirming that the patient was unwell was damaging to the patient's health or if patients suffered by being under-treated because of the coarseness of the clinical judgement possessed by the magistrates. Both these possible consequences of the old methods, particularly that concerning failure to treat, were real and serious. The architects of the Act chose to prevent them by by-passing magisterial intervention. Under the new provisions patients may be admitted for treatment on the application of the nearest relative or a mental welfare officer, if two medical practitioners (one preferably the patient's usual doctor and the other a psychiatrist) recommend the admission and if the grounds stated are sufficient; these must be that the patient is suffering from mental illness or severe subnormality, or, in the case of a patient under the age of twenty-one, alternative grounds that the person is suffering from psychopathic disorder.

This type of compulsory order (Admission for Treatment Order, Section 26) has a duration of one year in the first instance and is the most formal of the admission methods. It requires that the grounds for the medical opinions be stated on the forms, and is used when someone acknowledged to be ill can be committed at a dignified pace. Needless to say, the fact that the order lasts for a year in the first instance, and is then renewable for another year and thenceforth further renewable at two-year intervals, does not mean that it represents the imposition of any kind of fixed sentence; usually patients on orders recover insight rather quickly after entering hospital, and as soon as this happens the patient is likely to agree to stay in hospital voluntarily, whereupon the order is terminated.

Though the patient, having refused to enter hospital and having had an order made out, has no further say in the matter until he is in hospital, he may then apply to the local Mental Health Review Tribunal for redress and discharge and, if he does not obtain these, may reapply at intervals. The tribunal, composed of medical and legal members, and independent of the hospital, has the power to order the patient's discharge if he makes out a plausible case. Patients may also obtain their discharge by persuading the nearest relative to rescind his original application, by attaining the age of twenty-five (in the case of those suffering from psychopathic disorder, who may not be detained under this section after that age) or by escaping, when following a period of liberty varying according to the diagnostic category (six months for a psychopath, for example, and twenty-eight days for the mentally ill) the order automatically lapses.

By far the commonest method by which the order is terminated is that consequent upon complete or partial recovery, and the danger that patients might be kept against their will and without justification must, taking into account the overcrowded hospitals and the psychiatrists' eagerness to discharge, be a theoretical one. Not so theoretical, however, that special provisions for Members of Parliament were not incorporated in the Act, lest a pair of unscrupulous psychiatrists should compulsorily admit the Government on more or less defensible grounds (such as those of seriously irresponsible conduct) and achieve a *coup d'état*. The ease with which compulsory admission could be ordered under the new arrangements and the contrasting existence of special safeguards for Members of Parliament caused some disquiet among those conscious of the heritage of freedom, seeming as they did to presage a return to the eighteenth century concept of liberty, in which institutions rather than individuals were free. All laws depend in the end on the way in which they are applied, however, and this one is being used cautiously at present; but obviously the liberty of the individual must continue to be guarded alertly by the courts and legislature.

Where it is not certain that the patient is likely to need prolonged treatment or, as is more often the case, where the diagnosis cannot be made with any precision or detailed grounds for the advisability of admission stated, an unwilling patient may be admitted for a shorter period, for observation. Under the provisions of the relevant Sections (25 and 29) any form of mental disorder constitutes the grounds for such an admission, which means that not only minors but, under these sections, someone of more than twenty-one years of age can be admitted against his will solely on the grounds of psychopathic disorder (which under Section 26 he cannot) in order that he may be observed to see what lies behind his disturbance and whether treatment can help him. Admission for Observation in Case of

Emergency is an abbreviated procedure, when any relative or the Mental Welfare Officer may apply and any single doctor can recommend, the order lasting only for three days. Admission for Observation under Section 25, on the other hand, allows for the detention to continue for one month if need be.

This means that in theory it is now possible to detain in hospital adult patients whose conduct is abnormally aggressive or seriously irresponsible; presumably the Act makes it feasible to treat by this means the unwilling patients who are alcoholics, addicts, or prize delinquents. Attempts have been made in the past to bring these groups within the province of the psychiatrist by compulsory measures, but they have always failed. Probably psychiatrists are somewhat more able now to deal with these conditions, if indeed they all are conditions in the pathological sense, than they once were. But the Act has not been fully exploited, though it was intended that it should be, to bring treatment to alcoholics, drug-addicts, and the abnormally aggressive because there are, as yet, very few facilities for dealing with the special management problems these patients cause. They seldom fit into the routine of an ordinary mental hospital, and specialized units for them are mostly in the early planning stage. Also, because of the years of consideration of the legal concept of 'certifiability', psychiatrists are as unwilling as other citizens to take away the liberty of patients whose conduct is only quantitatively different from that shown by the general public and, when alone or in the company of one another, by the sanest of the psychiatrists themselves. When more can be offered to the patients suffering from psychopathic disorder in the way of specific measures the provisions for their compulsory admission may be used more often.

Part v of the Act deals with the role of the mental hospital in the treatment of criminal offenders. Obviously many patients whose illnesses are so severe as to make them unable to recognize or understand the social and legal requirements of the country in which they live fall foul of the law. Usually they do not go to court, because their abnormality is obvious, and admission to hospital is arranged straight away. Some of these patients may not be obviously ill at the time they are apprehended, or the importance of their illness in the causation of their illegal conduct is not sufficiently clear (particularly when a gainful crime has been committed) and they are tried. Usually the existence of psychosis is regarded as indicating treatment rather than punishment. Under Section 60 of the Act such offenders, or offenders with lesser psychiatric abnormalities than psychosis, can be committed to a mental hospital in lieu of imprisonment. The patient, once in hospital, is in the same position as someone under an Admission for Treatment Order, unless the Court has made a further stipulation restricting discharge. An Assize Court or Quarter Sessions may restrict the patient's discharge and indeed may do so without limit of time, when the order amounts to 'Her Majesty's pleasure'.

The linking of hospitals with courts in this way is welcome. At one time psychiatrically ill offenders were often sent to prison because they needed some kind of care, even though they did not, by virtue of their lack of responsibility for their actions, merit punishment: the courts were unable to order psychiatric treatment in prison and though pious hopes were expressed that the prisoners might obtain it the facilities were, as they remain, inadequate. On the other hand, speaking still of the days before the Act, the court could not arrange that the offender received psychiatric in-patient treatment if he were not certifiable except by making it a condition of probation, which meant recording a conviction and which, at all events, could not be extended longer than one year. The provision of Section 60 enables the courts to attain in some respects their aim of doing what is most appropriate for those that come before them.

The patients who may be committed under Section 60 include those with psychopathic disorder (in this instance, of any age). At present, as indicated previously, few psychiatrists and fewer hospitals can offer much to these patients, and even those hospitals that are willing to try to manage compulsorily detained psychopathic patients find that one or two such patients set their open-door and therapeutic-community plans back disproportionately and therefore sharply limit their numbers. The provisions are there for future use, and will be more frequently applied to psychopathic patients if and when their medical management improves or the Minister sets up new Special Hospitals (as Broadmoor, Rampton, and Moss Side are now called) for their detention.

Part VIII of the Act deals with the management of the property and affairs of patients whose illness renders them psychologically incompetent to conduct their own business. The Court of Protection may find, after hearing medical evidence, that a patient is mentally incapable of management and administration and order that his dependants are looked after, his estate maintained in a fair way, and both legal and unenforceable debts paid. Subsequently a receiver may be appointed to look after the business affairs. These provisions are of great assistance to relatives if the patient's estate is substantial and being badly or unfairly administered, and it is not necessary that the patient should be in hospital for the Court of Protection to intervene.

Part IX concerns miscellaneous topics and induces protective clauses, so important to those working in psychiatry, limiting the liability of those acting in good faith and with reasonable care and thereby reducing the shadow of litigation and enabling the psychiatrist and mental welfare officer to do their best for the patient without considering self-preservation.

The sweeping reforms of this Act have put Great Britain at the forefront of the world in the legal provision for the mentally disordered. The Act not only humanizes and simplifies the admission of patients, but makes procedures much more flexible so that future improvements in diagnosis and treatment can be fitted into the existing framework. The decision about compulsory admission is now largely in the hands of those expert in psychiatric illness, and in this way patients may, if necessary, be admitted in order to forestall inevitable permanent deterioration; it is expected that as the psychiatrists' capacity to treat effectively in this way increases, the reputation of psychiatry will further improve, and the need for compulsory measures diminish; already the proportion of patients in mental hospitals under orders has fallen from the majority to a small minority.

The principal theoretical reservation about the Act, a serious one, is the justifiability of depriving a resident of the United

Kingdom of his liberty without invoking a magistrate: in fact, quite apart from the reassuring observation, necessarily of uncertain value, that so far the powers have been used less rather than more than they should, the Mental Health Review Tribunals serve a magisterial function and do so more informally and informedly so that the patient, whether regarded as a sick man or a citizen possibly under duress, makes a gain in both roles. The principal practical disadvantage is that patients tend to leave hospital prematurely, exercising their rights under the informal admission procedures that prevail, so that many more of them, particularly the chronic schizophrenics, get into difficulties outside and need to be readmitted via the jails to which they are remanded.

Laws like the Mental Health Act (1959) are being framed and passed in many of the American States and in other countries of of the world; it remains for psychiatrists to justify the optimism shown by the legislators.

16   The Outlook

The standard at which psychiatry is practised depends principally on the thoroughness with which the subject is taught at
medical schools. The psychiatric training of medical practitioners is at present grossly deficient.

Even at the most favoured hospitals the student's experience with psychiatric patients, from which the most useful
teaching stems, is barely adequate; while at some teaching
hospitals the student scarcely sees a patient except at case-
demonstrations. The best students still manage to learn
enough psychiatry for their diagnostic needs, but the best
students are never the problem; the average or the weak
student needs ample case-work and instruction in small
groups, together with the stimulus of an examination in
psychiatry at the end of his training years, and he seldom gets
them.

There has recently been an increase in the number of chairs
of psychiatry in Britain and a reduction in the opposition to the
transfer of teaching time from gynaecology or surgery to
psychiatry, but much conservatism remains to be overcome and
the autonomy of the great hospitals makes it hard for governments to influence curricula except by the distasteful methods
of financial coercion; though the General Medical Council
could, if it wished, require that minimum standards in psychiatric skill be attained. Psychiatry has only recently become
respectable, if indeed the adjective is not still premature, and
some delay in full acceptance of the subject by the general
physicians and surgeons of the teaching hospitals is understandable; but the incorporation of the speciality into the
clinical curriculum with the status of an important part of the
whole should not be too long delayed because of the increasing

need for psychiatric knowledge in general practice as community services expand.

Even at its best, teaching-hospital psychiatry does not reflect the real problems that beset the doctor in general practice: the new undergraduate hospitals now being planned are based on communities, the aim being to provide a comprehensive hospital service for the sick of that community *with the exception of its psychiatric casualties*, of whom only a small proportion will receive treatment under the teaching hospital. Since these patients, particularly those who fail to recover completely, will form a sizeable proportion of the general practitioner's work load, any thorough training should include experience with them. Psychiatrists at teaching hospitals, having waged long campaigns to obtain a few beds, now find that their success is illusory; advances in management and treatment have made it necessary to incorporate long-stay psychiatric units, community mental-health organizations, and all the associated schemes into their departments if they are to maintain proper standards of care and teaching. The psychiatric departments envisaged for new teaching hospitals are already obsolete, and there is no sign that the planners are aware that this is the case.

Postgraduate training in psychiatry is somewhat uneven. Those who obtain posts at teaching hospitals are adequately tutored, though their experience in the treatment and management of long-stay patients will be slight. Those who train at the Institute of Psychiatry receive a comprehensive and systematic course covering important aspects of the speciality; but here again work with chronic patients is somewhat lacking. The doctors who work in junior posts in outlying hospitals see plenty of patients, long and short-stay, but they are seldom properly taught. The unpopularity of these very useful jobs, many of them filled by doctors from abroad and many of them not filled at all, is due in no small part to the poor provision that is made for case-discussion, formal study, and guidance in research. Thus the valuable experience available is largely wasted because of deficits that could be made good by Ministerial action. Because not more than a small percentage of psychiatrists can rotate from teaching hospital to postgraduate institute to mental hospital in order to maintain the correct balance in their experience, the main changes must be made in the mental hospitals: it is there that most trainee psychiatrists are employed. Some undergraduate teaching centres are starting interlocking schemes with their local mental hospitals, offering academic facilities and receiving a chance to look at the way the real work is done; the postgraduate Institute of Psychiatry, which has a reputation within the speciality for going its own divided way, is not looking outwards in a like manner.

Treatment advances in psychiatry may come, as so many have in the past, like bolts from the blue. Much of our knowledge about treatment still remains to be ordered and rationally applied, and for this, fortunately, geniuses are not required; only adequate numbers of psychiatrists with suitable facilities and funds, who may be marginally easier to come by.

In the long run the prospects for treatment in psychiatry depend on the development of the subject as a scientific study and for this the prospects are, in the long run, good. The blossoming of scientific psychology, in which the number of first-rate students graduating annually is many times greater than before the war and in which the powerful tools of computers and mathematical techniques have opened up the whole subject, means that soon we shall be provided with comparatively precise statements about the operations of the normal brain: a basis in normal psychology would revolutionize the whole study of psychiatry. I cannot predict what advances within psychiatry will shortly be made, nor say what specific areas are the most promising: however, much remains to be done before we can rely confidently even on our diagnostic schemes, and for my part I would like, if only as a first step, to see the disease entities more clearly separated and defined; not until this is done can the biochemical, epidemiological, sociological, and psychopathological studies make their full contribution to the speciality.

To a large extent the picture a doctor sees of his work consists of its deficiencies, since these make for the disappointments and the tragedies that occur despite his efforts. Even so, it is easy to end this review of the present state of psychiatry on a hopeful note. The variety and scope of the work being done is now immense and the small pools of knowledge are starting not only to spread but to coalesce, a process that can only accelerate as time goes by. For the young physician psychiatry has always offered the chance of intimate contact with the sick; recently it has conferred the respect of the majority of his colleagues; at present it gives the opportunity for much effective treatment and a vast choice of researches. It is a speciality of the future rather than the past.

Index

Italic figures indicate main references.

Some other Pelican books on psychology
are described on the following pages

Techniques of Persuasion
From Propaganda to Brainwashing

J. A. C. Brown

Attempts to change the opinions of others are as old as human speech, but in recent years we have come to fear that our thoughts and feelings are open to manipulation by new methods and hidden techniques. To the pressures of the 'admen' are added a whole battery of *hsi nao* (literally 'wash brain') techniques.

Here is a timely and much-needed survey of the whole area of persuasion. Dr Brown, the author of *Freud and the Post-Freudians,* ranges from political propaganda, religious conversion, and commercial advertising, through a detailed appraisal of the intentions and effects of the mass media, to a cool look at the spectacular case histories of indoctrination and confession.

But *Techniques of Persuasion* is more than the only available review of the phenomena of persuasion: it also contains a lucid analysis of the concept of personality itself. Only if we understand first the development of the central personality can we understand and judge realistically the importance of attempts to change it.

Also available:

THE SOCIAL PSYCHOLOGY OF INDUSTRY

Psychology in Pelicans

Pelican books have achieved an enviable reputation for publishing first-class books on psychology for the general reader. Among the titles available are:

Childhood and Adolescence *J. A. Hadfield*

Freud and the Post-Freudians *J. A. C. Brown*

Know Your Own I.Q. *and* Check Your Own I.Q.
Sense and Nonsense in Psychology *and* Uses and
Abuses of Psychology
H. J. Eysenck

The Normal Child and Some of His Abnormalities
C. W. Valentine

Introduction to Jung's Psychology *Frieda Fordham*

The Psychology of Perception *M. D. Vernon*

Also available in Penguins:

A Dictionary of Psychology *James Drever*

More Psychology in Pelicans

Among the other books on psychology published in Pelicans are:

Child Care and the Growth of Love *John Bowlby and Margaret Fry*

Human Groups *W. J. H. Sprott*

Memory, Facts and Fallacies *Ian M. L. Hunter*

Psychiatry To-day *David Stafford-Clark*

The Psychology of Sex *Oswald Schwarz*

The Psychology of Study *C. A. Mace*

The Psychology of Thinking *Robert Thomson*

Thinking to Some Purpose *Susan Stebbing*

Also available in Penguins:

Journey Through Adolescence *Doris Odlum*

Fundamentals of Psychology
C. J. Adcock

As publishers we recommend this new addition to the Pelican psychology series as a simple, logical, authoritative, and fair-minded introduction to psychology for all kinds of readers.

The author, who is a senior lecturer in New Zealand, has studied psychology both in England and in the United States. He approaches the study of human behaviour from the starting-point of our most primitive responses, the reflexes, which he explains simply in neurological terms. Illustrating his statements with concrete examples and with many instances from the most recent study of animal behaviour, he goes on to discuss our basic drives and needs, such as hunger, thirst, and the need for air, sleep, and security. His particular gift for advancing the reader's knowledge in easy stages allows him to explain the more complex workings of the autonomic nervous system and the processes of fear and anger, of learning, perception, and thinking, and of the patterning of personality in chapters which are as simple to comprehend as they are to read.

'Has succeeded in that most difficult task, the production of a good introductory text in psychology – *The Times Educational Supplement*

Sexual Deviation
Anthony Storr

This book is a brief account of the common types of
sexual behaviour which are generally considered
perverse or deviant, together with explanations of
their origins.

Sado-masochism, fetishism, and other types of sexual
deviation are often assumed by the public to be the
result of satiety or else of inordinate desire. It is not
generally understood that the unhappy compulsions
which plague the deviant person are evidence of an
inability to achieve normal sexual relationships,
and that such people deserve compassion rather than
condemnation.

In this new Pelican Anthony Storr, the author of *The
Integrity of the Personality*, shows how sexual
deviations can result from inner feelings of sexual
guilt and inferiority which have persisted from
childhood. This is within everybody's understanding
It may seem a far cry from the lover's pinch to the
whip of the sado-masochist, but embryonic forms of
even the most bizarre deviations can be shown to
exist in all of us.

Everyone who is interested in sex – and which of us
is not – will be interested in this authoritative
account, not only because it explains the sexual
feelings of others, but also because it illuminates
some of their own.

Also available:

THE INTEGRITY OF THE PERSONALITY

The Science of Animal Behaviour
P. L. Broadhurst

For generations men have employed dogs and hawks
to hunt, cormorants to fish, and performing animals
for entertainment. Modern research, on scientific
lines, may greatly widen the use of animals in human
society. In this brief and fascinating study the
director of the animal psychology laboratory at
London University's Institute of Psychiatry recounts
how, with the use of test apparatus, monkeys can
learn to work for wages paid in token coins; how
white rats can be trained to thread their way through
a maze or taught specific drills in such devices as the
'shuttle box'. He describes, too, the scientific
observations which have been made on the behaviour
in the wild of – for instance – penguins or crabs, and
the questions that these raise.

Such experimentation and observation, under
approved conditions, can be shown to advance the
treatment of human mental disorders and to help in
the study of such difficult problems as pre-natal
influences. The study of animal behaviour may also,
as the author suggests, lead to such extraordinary
developments as the training of chimpanzees as
engine-drivers or the employment of pigeons as
production-line inspectors.

This authoritative book explains very clearly the
meaning and purpose of modern research into animal
behaviour.

*For a complete list of books available please write to
Penguin Books whose address can be found
on the back of the title page*